THIS F*cking KETO DIET
Journal Belongs To:

_____

KETO BEFORE **& After**

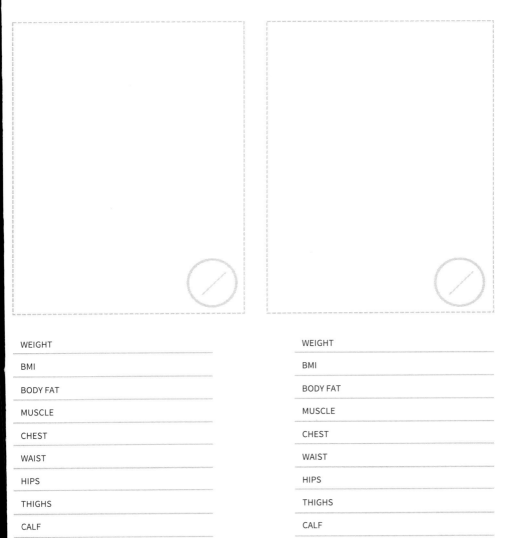

WEIGHT	WEIGHT
BMI	BMI
BODY FAT	BODY FAT
MUSCLE	MUSCLE
CHEST	CHEST
WAIST	WAIST
HIPS	HIPS
THIGHS	THIGHS
CALF	CALF
BICEP	BICEP
OTHER :	OTHER :
OTHER :	OTHER :

WEIGHT LOSS Start Date

*Describe what the hell I need to do to achieve my
most important health fitness goals.*

*I'm Tired of Feeling Sh*tty – How do I see
myself after I follow this Keto diet for 90 days?*

DATE	KETO WEIGHT LOSS ACTION PLAN		PERSONAL MILESTONES
		☐	
		☐	
		☐	
		☐	
		☐	
		☐	
		☐	
		☐	
		☐	
		☐	
		☐	
		☐	

Keto 15 Task Challenge

1 CREATE A KETO JOURNAL AND DOCUMENT YOUR PROGRESS COMPLETED ☐	**2** CHOOSE 7 KETO FRIENDLY RECIPES TO TRY COMPLETED ☐	**3** CREATE A WEEKLY MEAL PLANNER COMPLETED ☐
4 LOG EVERYTHING YOU EAT IN A WEIGHT LOSS APP COMPLETED ☐	**5** PURCHASE A FOOD SCALE AND SPIRALIZER COMPLETED ☐	**6** TRY BULLET PROOF COFFEE COMPLETED ☐
7 WEIGH YOURSELF EVERY WEEK COMPLETED ☐	**8** GO ALCOHOL FREE FOR ONE WEEK COMPLETED ☐	**9** TRY A 12-HOUR INTERMITTENT FAST COMPLETED ☐
10 CHECK AND LOG YOUR BODY MEASUREMENTS COMPLETED ☐	**11** LIST ALL THE REASONS WHY KETO WILL WORK FOR YOU COMPLETED ☐	**12** LEARN TO MAKE FAT BOMBS COMPLETED ☐
13 MONITOR YOUR WATER INTAKE COMPLETED ☐	**14** INCREASE YOUR HEALTHY FAT INTAKE COMPLETED ☐	**15** TEST KETONE LEVELS USING STRIPS COMPLETED ☐

Ketogenic Foods

MEATS	VEGGIES	VEGGIES	FRUITS
Beef	Avocado	Cucumber	Blackberries
Sausage	Asparagus	Chards	Cranberries
Bacon	Argula	Bell Peppers	Blueberries
Lamb	Broccoli	Green Beans	Lemon
Pork	Cauliflower	Collards	Lime
Veal	Brussel Sprouts	Mushrooms	Raspberries
Chicken/Turkey	Cabbage	Spinach	Strawberries
Eggs	Celery	Olives	Plantains (paleo)

DAIRY	CONDIMENTS	OILS & FATS	HERBS & SPICES
Cheese (all kinds)	Balsamic Vinegar	Avocado Oil	Garlic
Sour Cream	Beef/Chicken Broth	Butter	Salt & Pepper
Cream Cheese	Bonito Flakes	Coconut Butter	Oregano
Heavy Cream	Tartar Sauce (keto)	Duck Fat	Paprika
Greek Yogurt	Dijon Mustard	Lard/Ghee	Cumin
Almond Milk	Mayo	Nut Oils	Chili Pepper
Cashew Milk	Low Sugar Ketchup	Olive Oil	Basil
Coconut Cream	Pickles	Pork Rinds	Ginger

BAKING	FISH/SEAFOOD	DRINKS	MISC.
Almond Flour	Anchovy	Diet Soda (moderation)	Canned Tuna
Almond Meal	Haddock / Cod	Coffee	Pesto
Cashew Flour	Halibut	Tea	Soy Sauce
Oat Fiber	Crab/Lobster	Gatorade Zero	Aioli
Psyllium Husk	Mackerel	Protein Shake	Béarnaise
Whey Protein	Salmon	Club Soda	Vinaigrette
Flax meal	Tuna	Broth	Hot Sauce
Hazelnut Flour	Red Snapper	Coconut Water	Guacamole

NOTES:

Low Carb Grocery IDEAS

FRESH PRODUCE

☐ Asparagus	☐ Cauliflower	☐ Onions
☐ Avocado	☐ Celery	☐ Radishes
☐ Bell Peppers	☐ Cucumber	☐ Salad Mix
☐ Berries	☐ Eggplant	☐ Squash
☐ Broccoli	☐ Fennel	☐ Tomatoes
☐ Brussel Sprouts	☐ Garlic	☐ Bok Choi
☐ Cabbage	☐ Green Beans	☐ Chives
☐ Carrots	☐ Mushrooms	☐ Spinach

MEAT AND SEAFOOD

☐ Bacon	☐ Lamb	☐ Fish
☐ Beef	☐ Pork	☐ Crab
☐ Bison	☐ Rotisserie Chicken	☐ Lobster
☐ Chicken	☐ Sausage	☐ Scallops
☐ Deli meat	☐ Turkey	☐ Shrimp
☐ Ground Beef / Ground Turkey	☐ Oyster	☐ Mussels

DAIRY PRODUCTS

☐ Butter	☐ Eggs	☐ Sour Cream
☐ Cheese	☐ Greek Yogurt, full fat	☐ Ghee
☐ Cream Cheese	☐ Heavy Whipping Cream	☐ Mayo

PANTRY ITEMS

☐ Avocado oil	☐ Tea/Coffee	☐ Moon Cheese
☐ Beef Jerky	☐ Pork Rinds	☐ Low Carb Protein Bars
☐ Bone Broth	☐ Mayonnaise	☐ All Natural Peanut Butter
☐ Tuna, Salmon (canned)	☐ Low Carb Salad Dressing	☐ Stevia
☐ Coconut Butter	☐ Olive oil, extra virgin	☐ Almonds
☐ Coconut Oil	☐ Olives	☐ Spices
☐ Almond Milk	☐ Sweeteners	☐ Almond Flour

FROZEN / OTHER

☐	☐	☐
☐	☐	☐
☐	☐	☐
☐	☐	☐

My KETO GO TO **Meals**

KETO-FRIENDLY MEALS I'D DIE FOR (OR MAYBE THEY'RE JUST SIMPLE TO MAKE)

BREAKFAST	LUNCH	DINNER	SNACKS
BREAKFAST	LUNCH	DINNER	SNACKS
BREAKFAST	LUNCH	DINNER	SNACKS
BREAKFAST	LUNCH	DINNER	SNACKS
BREAKFAST	LUNCH	DINNER	SNACKS
BREAKFAST	LUNCH	DINNER	SNACKS
BREAKFAST	LUNCH	DINNER	SNACKS

MONTH BY MONTH **Tracker**

MONTHLY WEIGHT LOSS TRACKER TO TRACK WHAT THE HELL I'M DOING

JANUARY	JULY

FEBRUARY	AUGUST

MARCH	SEPTEMBER

APRIL	OCTOBER

MAY	NOVEMBER

JUNE	DECEMBER

MILESTONES	NOTES & REFLECTIONS

WEIGHT LOSS **Tracker**

WEEKLY WEIGHT LOSS TRACKER – Let's Get This SH*T Done!

MONTHLY GOAL

DATE:

	BUST				
	WAIST				
	HIPS				
	BICEP				
	THIGH				
	CALF				
	WEIGHT				
TOTAL WEIGHT LOSS >>					

INTERMITTENT **Fasting Log**

WEEK OF:

	START TIME	END TIME	TOTAL FAST HRS
M	:	:	:
T	:	:	:
W	:	:	:
T	:	:	:
F	:	:	:
S	:	:	:
S	:	:	:

WEEK OF:

	START TIME	END TIME	TOTAL FAST HRS
M	:	:	:
T	:	:	:
W	:	:	:
T	:	:	:
F	:	:	:
S	:	:	:
S	:	:	:

WEEK OF:

	START TIME	END TIME	TOTAL FAST HRS
M	:	:	:
T	:	:	:
W	:	:	:
T	:	:	:
F	:	:	:
S	:	:	:
S	:	:	:

WEEK OF:

	START TIME	END TIME	TOTAL FAST HRS
M	:	:	:
T	:	:	:
W	:	:	:
T	:	:	:
F	:	:	:
S	:	:	:
S	:	:	:

WEEK OF:

	START TIME	END TIME	TOTAL FAST HRS
M	:	:	:
T	:	:	:
W	:	:	:
T	:	:	:
F	:	:	:
S	:	:	:
S	:	:	:

MILESTONES & ACCOMPLISHMENTS

NOTES & REFLECTIONS

GOALS &
Accomplishments

THIS MONTH'S F*CKING GOALS

MY F*CKING ACTION PLAN   M T W T F S S

NOTES:

WEEKLY GOALS

THOUGHTS

MEAL IDEAS:	BREAKFAST	LUNCH	DINNER	SNACKS
M				
T				
W				
T				
F				
S				
S				

MEAL **Planner**

WEEK OF

GROCERY LIST

- [ ]
- [ ]
- [ ]
- [ ]
- [ ]
- [ ]
- [ ]
- [ ]
- [ ]
- [ ]
- [ ]
- [ ]
- [ ]
- [ ]
- [ ]
- [ ]
- [ ]
- [ ]

MON

TUES

WED

THUR

FRI

SAT

SUN

Low Carb Shopping List

FRESH PRODUCE

MEAT AND SEAFOOD

DAIRY PRODUCTS

PANTRY ITEMS

FROZEN / OTHER

I MAKE PROGRESS EVERY **Day**

SLEEP TRACKER:

DATE _____

☼ | RISE: | ☾ zᶻᶻ | BEDTIME: | zᶻᶻ | SLEEP (HRS):

MY NOTES FOR THE DAY

_____
_____
_____
_____

FASTING TIMES & DURATION

EXERCISE / WORKOUT ROUTINE

SLAY the DAY! – MY TOP 6 PRIORITIES

- ○ _____ ○ _____
- ○ _____ ○ _____
- ○ _____ ○ _____

IN A STATE OF KETOSIS?

YES   NO   UNSURE

WATER INTAKE TRACKER

DAILY ENERGY LEVEL

F*CKING GREAT	OKAY	SH*TTY

BREAKFAST

FAT: CARBS: PROTEIN: CALORIES:

LUNCH

FAT: CARBS: PROTEIN: CALORIES:

DINNER

FAT: CARBS: PROTEIN: CALORIES:

SNACKS

FAT: CARBS: PROTEIN: CALORIES:

END OF THE DAY TOTAL OVERVIEW

FAT	CARBS	PROTEIN	KCAL

I MAKE PROGRESS EVERY **Day**

SLEEP TRACKER:

DATE _____

☼ | RISE: | 🌙 zᶻᶻ | BEDTIME: | 💤 | SLEEP (HRS):

MY NOTES FOR THE DAY

_____

_____

_____

IN A STATE OF KETOSIS?

YES   NO   UNSURE

WATER INTAKE TRACKER

FASTING TIMES & DURATION

DAILY ENERGY LEVEL

F*CKING GREAT   OKAY   SH*TTY

BREAKFAST

FAT: CARBS: PROTEIN: CALORIES:

EXERCISE / WORKOUT ROUTINE

LUNCH

FAT: CARBS: PROTEIN: CALORIES:

DINNER

FAT: CARBS: PROTEIN: CALORIES:

SNACKS

FAT: CARBS: PROTEIN: CALORIES:

SLAY the DAY! – MY TOP 6 PRIORITIES

- ○
- ○
- ○
- ○
- ○
- ○

END OF THE DAY TOTAL OVERVIEW

FAT   CARBS   PROTEIN   KCAL

I MAKE PROGRESS EVERY **Day**

SLEEP TRACKER:

DATE _____

☀ RISE: _____ 🌙 BEDTIME: _____ 💤 SLEEP (HRS): _____

MY NOTES FOR THE DAY	IN A STATE OF KETOSIS?

IN A STATE OF KETOSIS?

YES   NO   UNSURE

WATER INTAKE TRACKER

💧 💧 💧 💧 💧 💧 💧 💧

FASTING TIMES & DURATION

DAILY ENERGY LEVEL		
F*CKING GREAT	OKAY	SH*TTY

BREAKFAST

FAT: CARBS: PROTEIN: CALORIES:

EXERCISE / WORKOUT ROUTINE

LUNCH

FAT: CARBS: PROTEIN: CALORIES:

DINNER

FAT: CARBS: PROTEIN: CALORIES:

SNACKS

FAT: CARBS: PROTEIN: CALORIES:

SLAY the DAY! – MY TOP 6 PRIORITIES

○ _____ ○ _____
○ _____ ○ _____
○ _____ ○ _____

END OF THE DAY TOTAL OVERVIEW

FAT	CARBS	PROTEIN	KCAL

I MAKE PROGRESS EVERY **Day**

SLEEP TRACKER:

DATE _____

☀ RISE: _____   🌙 BEDTIME: _____   💭 SLEEP (HRS): _____

MY NOTES FOR THE DAY

_____

_____

_____

FASTING TIMES & DURATION

EXERCISE / WORKOUT ROUTINE

SLAY the DAY! – MY TOP 6 PRIORITIES

- ○ _____   ○ _____
- ○ _____   ○ _____
- ○ _____   ○ _____

IN A STATE OF KETOSIS?

YES   NO   UNSURE

WATER INTAKE TRACKER

💧 💧 💧 💧 💧 💧 💧 💧

DAILY ENERGY LEVEL

F*CKING GREAT   OKAY   SH*TTY

BREAKFAST

FAT: CARBS: PROTEIN: CALORIES:

LUNCH

FAT: CARBS: PROTEIN: CALORIES:

DINNER

FAT: CARBS: PROTEIN: CALORIES:

SNACKS

FAT: CARBS: PROTEIN: CALORIES:

END OF THE DAY TOTAL OVERVIEW

FAT	CARBS	PROTEIN	KCAL

I MAKE PROGRESS EVERY **Day**

SLEEP TRACKER:

DATE _____

☼ RISE: _____   ☾ᶻᶻᶻ BEDTIME: _____   💤 SLEEP (HRS): _____

MY NOTES FOR THE DAY

_____
_____
_____

FASTING TIMES & DURATION

EXERCISE / WORKOUT ROUTINE

SLAY the DAY! – MY TOP 6 PRIORITIES

- ⚬ _____   ⚬ _____
- ⚬ _____   ⚬ _____
- ⚬ _____   ⚬ _____

IN A STATE OF KETOSIS?

YES   NO   UNSURE

WATER INTAKE TRACKER

🫧 🫧 🫧 🫧 🫧 🫧 🫧 🫧

DAILY ENERGY LEVEL

F*CKING GREAT   OKAY   SH*TTY

BREAKFAST

FAT: CARBS: PROTEIN: CALORIES:

LUNCH

FAT: CARBS: PROTEIN: CALORIES:

DINNER

FAT: CARBS: PROTEIN: CALORIES:

SNACKS

FAT: CARBS: PROTEIN: CALORIES:

END OF THE DAY TOTAL OVERVIEW

FAT	CARBS	PROTEIN	KCAL

I MAKE PROGRESS EVERY **Day**

SLEEP TRACKER:

DATE _____

☀ | RISE: | 🌙 zᶻᶻ | BEDTIME: | 💭zᶻᶻ | SLEEP (HRS):

MY NOTES FOR THE DAY

_____
_____
_____

FASTING TIMES & DURATION

EXERCISE / WORKOUT ROUTINE

SLAY the DAY! – MY TOP 6 PRIORITIES

● _____ ● _____
● _____ ● _____
● _____ ● _____

IN A STATE OF KETOSIS?

YES   NO   UNSURE

WATER INTAKE TRACKER

💧 💧 💧 💧 💧 💧 💧

DAILY ENERGY LEVEL

F*CKING GREAT   OKAY   SH*TTY

BREAKFAST

FAT: CARBS: PROTEIN: CALORIES:

LUNCH

FAT: CARBS: PROTEIN: CALORIES:

DINNER

FAT: CARBS: PROTEIN: CALORIES:

SNACKS

FAT: CARBS: PROTEIN: CALORIES:

END OF THE DAY TOTAL OVERVIEW

FAT	CARBS	PROTEIN	KCAL

I MAKE PROGRESS EVERY **Day**

SLEEP TRACKER:

DATE _____

| RISE: | BEDTIME: | SLEEP (HRS): |

MY NOTES FOR THE DAY

_____
_____
_____

FASTING TIMES & DURATION

EXERCISE / WORKOUT ROUTINE

SLAY the DAY! – MY TOP 6 PRIORITIES

IN A STATE OF KETOSIS?

YES   NO   UNSURE

WATER INTAKE TRACKER

DAILY ENERGY LEVEL

| F*CKING GREAT | OKAY | SH*TTY |

BREAKFAST

FAT: CARBS: PROTEIN: CALORIES:

LUNCH

FAT: CARBS: PROTEIN: CALORIES:

DINNER

FAT: CARBS: PROTEIN: CALORIES:

SNACKS

FAT: CARBS: PROTEIN: CALORIES:

END OF THE DAY TOTAL OVERVIEW

FAT	CARBS	PROTEIN	KCAL

MEAL **Planner**

WEEK OF

GROCERY LIST

MON

TUES

WED

THUR

FRI

SAT

SUN

Low Carb Shopping List

FRESH PRODUCE

MEAT AND SEAFOOD

DAIRY PRODUCTS

PANTRY ITEMS

FROZEN / OTHER

I MAKE PROGRESS EVERY Day

DATE _____

RISE: _____   BEDTIME: _____   SLEEP (HRS): _____

MY NOTES FOR THE DAY

_____
_____
_____

IN A STATE OF KETOSIS?

YES   NO   UNSURE

WATER INTAKE TRACKER

FASTING TIMES & DURATION

DAILY ENERGY LEVEL

F*CKING GREAT   OKAY   SH*TTY

BREAKFAST

FAT: CARBS: PROTEIN: CALORIES:

EXERCISE / WORKOUT ROUTINE

LUNCH

FAT: CARBS: PROTEIN: CALORIES:

DINNER

FAT: CARBS: PROTEIN: CALORIES:

SNACKS

FAT: CARBS: PROTEIN: CALORIES:

SLAY the DAY! – MY TOP 6 PRIORITIES

○ _____   ○ _____
○ _____   ○ _____
○ _____   ○ _____

END OF THE DAY TOTAL OVERVIEW

FAT	CARBS	PROTEIN	KCAL

I MAKE PROGRESS EVERY **Day**

SLEEP TRACKER:

DATE _____

☼ RISE: _____   🌙 BEDTIME: _____   💤 SLEEP (HRS): _____

MY NOTES FOR THE DAY	IN A STATE OF KETOSIS?

_____

_____

	YES NO UNSURE

WATER INTAKE TRACKER

💧 💧 💧 💧 💧 💧 💧 💧 💧

FASTING TIMES & DURATION

DAILY ENERGY LEVEL		
F*CKING GREAT	**OKAY**	**SH*TTY**

BREAKFAST

FAT: CARBS: PROTEIN: CALORIES:

EXERCISE / WORKOUT ROUTINE

LUNCH

FAT: CARBS: PROTEIN: CALORIES:

DINNER

FAT: CARBS: PROTEIN: CALORIES:

SNACKS

FAT: CARBS: PROTEIN: CALORIES:

SLAY the DAY! – MY TOP 6 PRIORITIES

END OF THE DAY TOTAL OVERVIEW			
FAT	CARBS	PROTEIN	KCAL

⊙ _____   ⊙ _____
⊙ _____   ⊙ _____
⊙ _____   ⊙ _____

I MAKE PROGRESS EVERY Day

SLEEP TRACKER:

DATE _____

☀ RISE: _____   🌙 zᶻᶻ BEDTIME: _____   💭zᶻᶻ SLEEP (HRS): _____

MY NOTES FOR THE DAY

_____
_____
_____

FASTING TIMES & DURATION

EXERCISE / WORKOUT ROUTINE

SLAY the DAY! - MY TOP 6 PRIORITIES

- ⚬ _____   ⚬ _____
- ⚬ _____   ⚬ _____
- ⚬ _____   ⚬ _____

IN A STATE OF KETOSIS?

YES   NO   UNSURE

WATER INTAKE TRACKER

DAILY ENERGY LEVEL

F*CKING GREAT   OKAY   SH*TTY

BREAKFAST

FAT: CARBS: PROTEIN: CALORIES:

LUNCH

FAT: CARBS: PROTEIN: CALORIES:

DINNER

FAT: CARBS: PROTEIN: CALORIES:

SNACKS

FAT: CARBS: PROTEIN: CALORIES:

END OF THE DAY TOTAL OVERVIEW

FAT	CARBS	PROTEIN	KCAL

I MAKE PROGRESS EVERY **Day**

SLEEP TRACKER:

DATE _____

RISE: _____ BEDTIME: _____ SLEEP (HRS): _____

MY NOTES FOR THE DAY

_____

_____

_____

FASTING TIMES & DURATION

EXERCISE / WORKOUT ROUTINE

SLAY the DAY! – MY TOP 6 PRIORITIES

IN A STATE OF KETOSIS?

YES   NO   UNSURE

WATER INTAKE TRACKER

DAILY ENERGY LEVEL		
F*CKING GREAT	OKAY	SH*TTY

BREAKFAST

FAT: CARBS: PROTEIN: CALORIES:

LUNCH

FAT: CARBS: PROTEIN: CALORIES:

DINNER

FAT: CARBS: PROTEIN: CALORIES:

SNACKS

FAT: CARBS: PROTEIN: CALORIES:

END OF THE DAY TOTAL OVERVIEW

FAT	CARBS	PROTEIN	KCAL

I MAKE PROGRESS EVERY Day

SLEEP TRACKER:

DATE _____

RISE: [   ]   BEDTIME: [   ]   SLEEP (HRS): [   ]

MY NOTES FOR THE DAY

_____

_____

_____

FASTING TIMES & DURATION

EXERCISE / WORKOUT ROUTINE

SLAY the DAY! – MY TOP 6 PRIORITIES

- ○ _____   ○ _____
- ○ _____   ○ _____
- ○ _____   ○ _____

IN A STATE OF KETOSIS?

YES   NO   UNSURE

WATER INTAKE TRACKER

DAILY ENERGY LEVEL

F*CKING GREAT   OKAY   SH*TTY

BREAKFAST

FAT: CARBS: PROTEIN: CALORIES:

LUNCH

FAT: CARBS: PROTEIN: CALORIES:

DINNER

FAT: CARBS: PROTEIN: CALORIES:

SNACKS

FAT: CARBS: PROTEIN: CALORIES:

END OF THE DAY TOTAL OVERVIEW

FAT   CARBS   PROTEIN   KCAL

I MAKE PROGRESS EVERY **Day**

SLEEP TRACKER:

DATE _____

RISE: _____   BEDTIME: _____   SLEEP (HRS): _____

MY NOTES FOR THE DAY

_____

_____

_____

FASTING TIMES & DURATION

EXERCISE / WORKOUT ROUTINE

SLAY the DAY! – MY TOP 6 PRIORITIES

○ _____   ○ _____
○ _____   ○ _____
○ _____   ○ _____

IN A STATE OF KETOSIS?

YES   NO   UNSURE

WATER INTAKE TRACKER

DAILY ENERGY LEVEL

F*CKING GREAT	OKAY	SH*TTY

BREAKFAST

FAT: CARBS: PROTEIN: CALORIES:

LUNCH

FAT: CARBS: PROTEIN: CALORIES:

DINNER

FAT: CARBS: PROTEIN: CALORIES:

SNACKS

FAT: CARBS: PROTEIN: CALORIES:

END OF THE DAY TOTAL OVERVIEW

FAT	CARBS	PROTEIN	KCAL

I MAKE PROGRESS EVERY Day

SLEEP TRACKER:

DATE _____

RISE: _____   BEDTIME: _____   SLEEP (HRS): _____

MY NOTES FOR THE DAY

_____

_____

_____

FASTING TIMES & DURATION

EXERCISE / WORKOUT ROUTINE

SLAY the DAY! – MY TOP 6 PRIORITIES

- ○ _____   ○ _____
- ○ _____   ○ _____
- ○ _____   ○ _____

IN A STATE OF KETOSIS?

YES   NO   UNSURE

WATER INTAKE TRACKER

DAILY ENERGY LEVEL

F*CKING GREAT	OKAY	SH*TTY

BREAKFAST

FAT: CARBS: PROTEIN: CALORIES:

LUNCH

FAT: CARBS: PROTEIN: CALORIES:

DINNER

FAT: CARBS: PROTEIN: CALORIES:

SNACKS

FAT: CARBS: PROTEIN: CALORIES:

END OF THE DAY TOTAL OVERVIEW

FAT	CARBS	PROTEIN	KCAL

MEAL **Planner**

WEEK OF

GROCERY LIST

- ☐
- ☐
- ☐
- ☐
- ☐
- ☐
- ☐
- ☐
- ☐
- ☐
- ☐
- ☐
- ☐
- ☐
- ☐
- ☐
- ☐
- ☐

MON

TUES

WED

THUR

FRI

SAT

SUN

Low Carb Shopping List

FRESH PRODUCE

MEAT AND SEAFOOD

DAIRY PRODUCTS

PANTRY ITEMS

FROZEN / OTHER

I MAKE PROGRESS EVERY **Day**

SLEEP TRACKER:

DATE _____

RISE: _____

BEDTIME: _____

SLEEP (HRS): _____

MY NOTES FOR THE DAY

_____

_____

_____

FASTING TIMES & DURATION

EXERCISE / WORKOUT ROUTINE

SLAY the DAY! – MY TOP 6 PRIORITIES

IN A STATE OF KETOSIS?

YES   NO   UNSURE

WATER INTAKE TRACKER

DAILY ENERGY LEVEL		
F*CKING GREAT	OKAY	SH*TTY

BREAKFAST

FAT: CARBS: PROTEIN: CALORIES:

LUNCH

FAT: CARBS: PROTEIN: CALORIES:

DINNER

FAT: CARBS: PROTEIN: CALORIES:

SNACKS

FAT: CARBS: PROTEIN: CALORIES:

END OF THE DAY TOTAL OVERVIEW

FAT	CARBS	PROTEIN	KCAL

I MAKE PROGRESS EVERY Day

SLEEP TRACKER:

DATE _____

RISE: _____   BEDTIME: _____   SLEEP (HRS): _____

MY NOTES FOR THE DAY

_____
_____
_____

IN A STATE OF KETOSIS?

YES   NO   UNSURE

WATER INTAKE TRACKER

FASTING TIMES & DURATION

DAILY ENERGY LEVEL

F*CKING GREAT	OKAY	SH*TTY

BREAKFAST

FAT: CARBS: PROTEIN: CALORIES:

EXERCISE / WORKOUT ROUTINE

LUNCH

FAT: CARBS: PROTEIN: CALORIES:

DINNER

FAT: CARBS: PROTEIN: CALORIES:

SNACKS

FAT: CARBS: PROTEIN: CALORIES:

SLAY the DAY! – MY TOP 6 PRIORITIES

END OF THE DAY TOTAL OVERVIEW

FAT	CARBS	PROTEIN	KCAL

I MAKE PROGRESS EVERY **Day**

DATE _____

RISE: _____   BEDTIME: _____   SLEEP (HRS): _____

MY NOTES FOR THE DAY

_____
_____
_____

FASTING TIMES & DURATION

EXERCISE / WORKOUT ROUTINE

SLAY the DAY! – MY TOP 6 PRIORITIES

- ○
- ○
- ○

IN A STATE OF KETOSIS?

YES   NO   UNSURE

WATER INTAKE TRACKER

DAILY ENERGY LEVEL

F*CKING GREAT   **OKAY**   **SH*TTY**

BREAKFAST

FAT: CARBS: PROTEIN: CALORIES:

LUNCH

FAT: CARBS: PROTEIN: CALORIES:

DINNER

FAT: CARBS: PROTEIN: CALORIES:

SNACKS

FAT: CARBS: PROTEIN: CALORIES:

END OF THE DAY TOTAL OVERVIEW

FAT	CARBS	PROTEIN	KCAL

I MAKE PROGRESS EVERY Day

SLEEP TRACKER:

DATE _____

RISE: _____   BEDTIME: _____   SLEEP (HRS): _____

MY NOTES FOR THE DAY

_____

_____

_____

FASTING TIMES & DURATION

EXERCISE / WORKOUT ROUTINE

SLAY the DAY! – MY TOP 6 PRIORITIES

- _____   - _____
- _____   - _____
- _____   - _____

IN A STATE OF KETOSIS?

YES   NO   UNSURE

WATER INTAKE TRACKER

DAILY ENERGY LEVEL

F*CKING GREAT   OKAY   SH*TTY

BREAKFAST

FAT: CARBS: PROTEIN: CALORIES:

LUNCH

FAT: CARBS: PROTEIN: CALORIES:

DINNER

FAT: CARBS: PROTEIN: CALORIES:

SNACKS

FAT: CARBS: PROTEIN: CALORIES:

END OF THE DAY TOTAL OVERVIEW

FAT	CARBS	PROTEIN	KCAL

I MAKE PROGRESS EVERY **Day**

SLEEP TRACKER:

DATE _____

RISE: _____   BEDTIME: _____   SLEEP (HRS): _____

MY NOTES FOR THE DAY

_____
_____
_____

FASTING TIMES & DURATION

EXERCISE / WORKOUT ROUTINE

SLAY the DAY! – MY TOP 6 PRIORITIES

- ⚪ ⚪
- ⚪ ⚪
- ⚪ ⚪

IN A STATE OF KETOSIS?

YES   NO   UNSURE

WATER INTAKE TRACKER

💧 💧 💧 💧 💧 💧 💧 💧

DAILY ENERGY LEVEL		
F*CKING GREAT	OKAY	SH*TTY

BREAKFAST

FAT: CARBS: PROTEIN: CALORIES:

LUNCH

FAT: CARBS: PROTEIN: CALORIES:

DINNER

FAT: CARBS: PROTEIN: CALORIES:

SNACKS

FAT: CARBS: PROTEIN: CALORIES:

END OF THE DAY TOTAL OVERVIEW

FAT	CARBS	PROTEIN	KCAL

I MAKE PROGRESS EVERY **Day**

SLEEP TRACKER:

DATE _____

☀ RISE: _____   🌙 BEDTIME: _____   💤 SLEEP (HRS): _____

MY NOTES FOR THE DAY

_____
_____
_____

IN A STATE OF KETOSIS?

YES   NO   UNSURE

WATER INTAKE TRACKER

FASTING TIMES & DURATION

DAILY ENERGY LEVEL

F*CKING GREAT	OKAY	SH*TTY

BREAKFAST

FAT: CARBS: PROTEIN: CALORIES:

LUNCH

FAT: CARBS: PROTEIN: CALORIES:

EXERCISE / WORKOUT ROUTINE

DINNER

FAT: CARBS: PROTEIN: CALORIES:

SNACKS

FAT: CARBS: PROTEIN: CALORIES:

SLAY the DAY! – MY TOP 6 PRIORITIES

- ○ _____   ○ _____
- ○ _____   ○ _____
- ○ _____   ○ _____

END OF THE DAY TOTAL OVERVIEW

FAT	CARBS	PROTEIN	KCAL

I MAKE PROGRESS EVERY **Day**

SLEEP TRACKER:

DATE _____

☀ RISE: _____ 🌙 BEDTIME: _____ 💭 SLEEP (HRS): _____

MY NOTES FOR THE DAY

_____
_____
_____

FASTING TIMES & DURATION

EXERCISE / WORKOUT ROUTINE

SLAY the DAY! – MY TOP 6 PRIORITIES

IN A STATE OF KETOSIS?

YES   NO   UNSURE

WATER INTAKE TRACKER

💧 💧 💧 💧 💧 💧 💧 💧

DAILY ENERGY LEVEL

F*CKING GREAT   OKAY   SH*TTY

BREAKFAST

FAT: CARBS: PROTEIN: CALORIES:

LUNCH

FAT: CARBS: PROTEIN: CALORIES:

DINNER

FAT: CARBS: PROTEIN: CALORIES:

SNACKS

FAT: CARBS: PROTEIN: CALORIES:

END OF THE DAY TOTAL OVERVIEW

FAT	CARBS	PROTEIN	KCAL

MEAL Planner

WEEK OF

GROCERY LIST

☐
☐
☐
☐
☐
☐
☐
☐
☐
☐
☐
☐
☐
☐
☐
☐
☐
☐

MON

TUES

WED

THUR

FRI

SAT

SUN

Low Carb Shopping List

FRESH PRODUCE

MEAT AND SEAFOOD

DAIRY PRODUCTS

PANTRY ITEMS

FROZEN / OTHER

I MAKE PROGRESS EVERY Day

SLEEP TRACKER:

DATE _____

RISE: _____   BEDTIME: _____   SLEEP (HRS): _____

MY NOTES FOR THE DAY

_____

_____

_____

_____

FASTING TIMES & DURATION

EXERCISE / WORKOUT ROUTINE

SLAY the DAY! – MY TOP 6 PRIORITIES

- ○ _____   ○ _____
- ○ _____   ○ _____
- ○ _____   ○ _____

IN A STATE OF KETOSIS?

YES   NO   UNSURE

WATER INTAKE TRACKER

DAILY ENERGY LEVEL

F*CKING GREAT   OKAY   SH*TTY

BREAKFAST

FAT: CARBS: PROTEIN: CALORIES:

LUNCH

FAT: CARBS: PROTEIN: CALORIES:

DINNER

FAT: CARBS: PROTEIN: CALORIES:

SNACKS

FAT: CARBS: PROTEIN: CALORIES:

END OF THE DAY TOTAL OVERVIEW

FAT   CARBS   PROTEIN   KCAL

I MAKE PROGRESS EVERY **Day**

SLEEP TRACKER:

DATE _____

RISE: _____   BEDTIME: _____   SLEEP (HRS): _____

MY NOTES FOR THE DAY

_____
_____
_____

FASTING TIMES & DURATION

EXERCISE / WORKOUT ROUTINE

SLAY the DAY! – MY TOP 6 PRIORITIES

IN A STATE OF KETOSIS?

YES   NO   UNSURE

WATER INTAKE TRACKER

DAILY ENERGY LEVEL

F*CKING GREAT   OKAY   SH*TTY

BREAKFAST

FAT: CARBS: PROTEIN: CALORIES:

LUNCH

FAT: CARBS: PROTEIN: CALORIES:

DINNER

FAT: CARBS: PROTEIN: CALORIES:

SNACKS

FAT: CARBS: PROTEIN: CALORIES:

END OF THE DAY TOTAL OVERVIEW

FAT	CARBS	PROTEIN	KCAL

I MAKE PROGRESS EVERY **Day**

SLEEP TRACKER:

DATE _____

RISE: _____ BEDTIME: _____ SLEEP (HRS): _____

MY NOTES FOR THE DAY

_____
_____
_____

FASTING TIMES & DURATION

EXERCISE / WORKOUT ROUTINE

SLAY the DAY! – MY TOP 6 PRIORITIES

- _____   - _____
- _____   - _____
- _____   - _____

IN A STATE OF KETOSIS?

YES   NO   UNSURE

WATER INTAKE TRACKER

DAILY ENERGY LEVEL

F*CKING GREAT   OKAY   SH*TTY

BREAKFAST

FAT: CARBS: PROTEIN: CALORIES:

LUNCH

FAT: CARBS: PROTEIN: CALORIES:

DINNER

FAT: CARBS: PROTEIN: CALORIES:

SNACKS

FAT: CARBS: PROTEIN: CALORIES:

END OF THE DAY TOTAL OVERVIEW

FAT	CARBS	PROTEIN	KCAL

I MAKE PROGRESS EVERY **Day**

SLEEP TRACKER:

DATE _____

RISE: | BEDTIME: | SLEEP (HRS):

MY NOTES FOR THE DAY

_____

_____

_____

IN A STATE OF KETOSIS?

YES   NO   UNSURE

WATER INTAKE TRACKER

FASTING TIMES & DURATION

DAILY ENERGY LEVEL		
F*CKING GREAT	**OKAY**	**SH*TTY**

BREAKFAST

FAT: CARBS: PROTEIN: CALORIES:

LUNCH

FAT: CARBS: PROTEIN: CALORIES:

EXERCISE / WORKOUT ROUTINE

DINNER

FAT: CARBS: PROTEIN: CALORIES:

SNACKS

FAT: CARBS: PROTEIN: CALORIES:

SLAY the DAY! – MY TOP 6 PRIORITIES

END OF THE DAY TOTAL OVERVIEW

FAT   CARBS   PROTEIN   KCAL

I MAKE PROGRESS EVERY **Day**

SLEEP TRACKER:

RISE: _____   BEDTIME: _____   SLEEP (HRS): _____

MY NOTES FOR THE DAY

_____
_____
_____

IN A STATE OF KETOSIS?

YES   NO   UNSURE

WATER INTAKE TRACKER

FASTING TIMES & DURATION

DAILY ENERGY LEVEL

F*CKING GREAT   OKAY   SH*TTY

BREAKFAST

FAT: CARBS: PROTEIN: CALORIES:

EXERCISE / WORKOUT ROUTINE

LUNCH

FAT: CARBS: PROTEIN: CALORIES:

DINNER

FAT: CARBS: PROTEIN: CALORIES:

SNACKS

FAT: CARBS: PROTEIN: CALORIES:

SLAY the DAY! – MY TOP 6 PRIORITIES

- ⦿ _____   ⦿ _____
- ⦿ _____   ⦿ _____
- ⦿ _____   ⦿ _____

END OF THE DAY TOTAL OVERVIEW

FAT	CARBS	PROTEIN	KCAL

I MAKE PROGRESS EVERY **Day**

SLEEP TRACKER:

DATE _____

RISE: _____

🌙 ᶻᶻᶻ BEDTIME: _____

💤 SLEEP (HRS): _____

MY NOTES FOR THE DAY

_____

_____

_____

FASTING TIMES & DURATION

EXERCISE / WORKOUT ROUTINE

SLAY the DAY! – MY TOP 6 PRIORITIES

- ○ _____ ○ _____
- ○ _____ ○ _____
- ○ _____ ○ _____

IN A STATE OF KETOSIS?

YES   NO   UNSURE

WATER INTAKE TRACKER

💧 💧 💧 💧 💧 💧 💧 💧

DAILY ENERGY LEVEL		
F*CKING GREAT	OKAY	SH*TTY

BREAKFAST

FAT: CARBS: PROTEIN: CALORIES:

LUNCH

FAT: CARBS: PROTEIN: CALORIES:

DINNER

FAT: CARBS: PROTEIN: CALORIES:

SNACKS

FAT: CARBS: PROTEIN: CALORIES:

END OF THE DAY TOTAL OVERVIEW

FAT	CARBS	PROTEIN	KCAL

I MAKE PROGRESS EVERY **Day**

SLEEP TRACKER:

DATE _____

RISE: _____   BEDTIME: _____   SLEEP (HRS): _____

MY NOTES FOR THE DAY
_____
_____
_____
_____

IN A STATE OF KETOSIS?

YES   NO   UNSURE

WATER INTAKE TRACKER

FASTING TIMES & DURATION

DAILY ENERGY LEVEL

F*CKING GREAT   OKAY   SH*TTY

BREAKFAST

FAT: CARBS: PROTEIN: CALORIES:

LUNCH

FAT: CARBS: PROTEIN: CALORIES:

EXERCISE / WORKOUT ROUTINE

DINNER

FAT: CARBS: PROTEIN: CALORIES:

SNACKS

FAT: CARBS: PROTEIN: CALORIES:

SLAY the DAY! – MY TOP 6 PRIORITIES

- _____   _____
- _____   _____
- _____   _____

END OF THE DAY TOTAL OVERVIEW

FAT   CARBS   PROTEIN   KCAL

MEAL **Planner**

GROCERY LIST

- ☐
- ☐
- ☐
- ☐
- ☐
- ☐
- ☐
- ☐
- ☐
- ☐
- ☐
- ☐
- ☐
- ☐
- ☐
- ☐
- ☐
- ☐

MON

TUES

WED

THUR

FRI

SAT

SUN

Low Carb Shopping List

FRESH PRODUCE

MEAT AND SEAFOOD

DAIRY PRODUCTS

PANTRY ITEMS

FROZEN / OTHER

I MAKE PROGRESS EVERY **Day**

SLEEP TRACKER:

DATE _____

RISE: _____

BEDTIME: _____

SLEEP (HRS): _____

MY NOTES FOR THE DAY

_____

_____

_____

FASTING TIMES & DURATION

EXERCISE / WORKOUT ROUTINE

IN A STATE OF KETOSIS?

YES   NO   UNSURE

WATER INTAKE TRACKER

DAILY ENERGY LEVEL

F*CKING GREAT	OKAY	SH*TTY

BREAKFAST

FAT: CARBS: PROTEIN: CALORIES:

LUNCH

FAT: CARBS: PROTEIN: CALORIES:

DINNER

FAT: CARBS: PROTEIN: CALORIES:

SNACKS

FAT: CARBS: PROTEIN: CALORIES:

SLAY the DAY! – MY TOP 6 PRIORITIES

END OF THE DAY TOTAL OVERVIEW

FAT	CARBS	PROTEIN	KCAL

I MAKE PROGRESS EVERY **Day**

SLEEP TRACKER:

RISE: _____

BEDTIME: _____

SLEEP (HRS): _____

MY NOTES FOR THE DAY

_____
_____
_____

FASTING TIMES & DURATION

EXERCISE / WORKOUT ROUTINE

SLAY the DAY! – MY TOP 6 PRIORITIES

- ⦾ _____   ⦾ _____
- ⦾ _____   ⦾ _____
- ⦾ _____   ⦾ _____

IN A STATE OF KETOSIS?

YES   NO   UNSURE

WATER INTAKE TRACKER

DAILY ENERGY LEVEL		
F*CKING GREAT	OKAY	SH*TTY

BREAKFAST

FAT: CARBS: PROTEIN: CALORIES:

LUNCH

FAT: CARBS: PROTEIN: CALORIES:

DINNER

FAT: CARBS: PROTEIN: CALORIES:

SNACKS

FAT: CARBS: PROTEIN: CALORIES:

END OF THE DAY TOTAL OVERVIEW

FAT	CARBS	PROTEIN	KCAL

WEIGHT LOSS **Tracker**

WEEKLY WEIGHT LOSS TRACKER – Let's Get This SH*T Done!

MONTHLY GOAL

_____

DATE: _____ _____ _____ _____ _____

	BUST				
	WAIST				
	HIPS				
	BICEP				
	THIGH				
	CALF				
	WEIGHT				
TOTAL WEIGHT LOSS >>					

INTERMITTENT Fasting Log

WEEK OF:

	START TIME	END TIME	TOTAL FAST HRS
M	:	:	:
T	:	:	:
W	:	:	:
T	:	:	:
F	:	:	:
S	:	:	:
S	:	:	:

WEEK OF:

	START TIME	END TIME	TOTAL FAST HRS
M	:	:	:
T	:	:	:
W	:	:	:
T	:	:	:
F	:	:	:
S	:	:	:
S	:	:	:

WEEK OF:

	START TIME	END TIME	TOTAL FAST HRS
M	:	:	:
T	:	:	:
W	:	:	:
T	:	:	:
F	:	:	:
S	:	:	:
S	:	:	:

WEEK OF:

	START TIME	END TIME	TOTAL FAST HRS
M	:	:	:
T	:	:	:
W	:	:	:
T	:	:	:
F	:	:	:
S	:	:	:
S	:	:	:

WEEK OF:

	START TIME	END TIME	TOTAL FAST HRS
M	:	:	:
T	:	:	:
W	:	:	:
T	:	:	:
F	:	:	:
S	:	:	:
S	:	:	:

NOTES & REFLECTIONS

MILESTONES & ACCOMPLISHMENTS

GOALS &
Accomplishments

MONTH | JAN FEB MAR APR MAY JUN JUL AUG SEP OCT NOV DEC

THIS MONTH'S F*CKING GOALS

_____   _____
_____   _____
_____   _____

MY F*CKING ACTION PLAN

M T W T F S S

☐ ☐ ☐ ☐ ☐ ☐ ☐
☐ ☐ ☐ ☐ ☐ ☐ ☐
☐ ☐ ☐ ☐ ☐ ☐ ☐
☐ ☐ ☐ ☐ ☐ ☐ ☐
☐ ☐ ☐ ☐ ☐ ☐ ☐

NOTES:

WEEKLY GOALS

THOUGHTS

MEAL IDEAS:	BREAKFAST	LUNCH	DINNER	SNACKS
M				
T				
W				
T				
F				
S				
S				

I MAKE PROGRESS EVERY **Day**

SLEEP TRACKER:

DATE _____

☀ RISE: _____   🌙 z,z,z BEDTIME: _____   💭zzz SLEEP (HRS): _____

MY NOTES FOR THE DAY

_____

_____

_____

FASTING TIMES & DURATION

EXERCISE / WORKOUT ROUTINE

SLAY the DAY! – MY TOP 6 PRIORITIES

⦿ _____   ⦿ _____

⦿ _____   ⦿ _____

⦿ _____   ⦿ _____

IN A STATE OF KETOSIS?

YES   NO   UNSURE

WATER INTAKE TRACKER

💧 💧 💧 💧 💧 💧 💧 💧

DAILY ENERGY LEVEL

F*CKING GREAT	OKAY	SH*TTY

BREAKFAST

FAT: CARBS: PROTEIN: CALORIES:

LUNCH

FAT: CARBS: PROTEIN: CALORIES:

DINNER

FAT: CARBS: PROTEIN: CALORIES:

SNACKS

FAT: CARBS: PROTEIN: CALORIES:

END OF THE DAY TOTAL OVERVIEW

FAT	CARBS	PROTEIN	KCAL

I MAKE PROGRESS EVERY **Day**

SLEEP TRACKER:

DATE _____

RISE: _____ | BEDTIME: _____ | SLEEP (HRS): _____

MY NOTES FOR THE DAY

_____
_____
_____

FASTING TIMES & DURATION

EXERCISE / WORKOUT ROUTINE

SLAY the DAY! – MY TOP 6 PRIORITIES

- ● _____ ● _____
- ● _____ ● _____
- ● _____ ● _____

IN A STATE OF KETOSIS?

YES   NO   UNSURE

WATER INTAKE TRACKER

DAILY ENERGY LEVEL

F*CKING GREAT	OKAY	SH*TTY

BREAKFAST

FAT: CARBS: PROTEIN: CALORIES:

LUNCH

FAT: CARBS: PROTEIN: CALORIES:

DINNER

FAT: CARBS: PROTEIN: CALORIES:

SNACKS

FAT: CARBS: PROTEIN: CALORIES:

END OF THE DAY TOTAL OVERVIEW

FAT	CARBS	PROTEIN	KCAL

I MAKE PROGRESS EVERY Day

DATE _____

| RISE: | BEDTIME: | SLEEP (HRS): |

MY NOTES FOR THE DAY

_____

_____

_____

FASTING TIMES & DURATION

EXERCISE / WORKOUT ROUTINE

SLAY the DAY! – MY TOP 6 PRIORITIES

- ○ _____   ○ _____
- ○ _____   ○ _____
- ○ _____   ○ _____

IN A STATE OF KETOSIS?

YES   NO   UNSURE

WATER INTAKE TRACKER

DAILY ENERGY LEVEL

F*CKING GREAT   OKAY   SH*TTY

BREAKFAST

FAT: CARBS: PROTEIN: CALORIES:

LUNCH

FAT: CARBS: PROTEIN: CALORIES:

DINNER

FAT: CARBS: PROTEIN: CALORIES:

SNACKS

FAT: CARBS: PROTEIN: CALORIES:

END OF THE DAY TOTAL OVERVIEW

FAT	CARBS	PROTEIN	KCAL

I MAKE PROGRESS EVERY **Day**

SLEEP TRACKER:

DATE _____

☀ RISE: _____   🌙 z$_z$^{z} BEDTIME: _____   💭 z^{z}z SLEEP (HRS): _____

MY NOTES FOR THE DAY

_____
_____

FASTING TIMES & DURATION

EXERCISE / WORKOUT ROUTINE

IN A STATE OF KETOSIS?

YES   NO   UNSURE

WATER INTAKE TRACKER

💧 💧 💧 💧 💧 💧 💧 💧

DAILY ENERGY LEVEL		
F*CKING GREAT	OKAY	SH*TTY

BREAKFAST

FAT: CARBS: PROTEIN: CALORIES:

LUNCH

FAT: CARBS: PROTEIN: CALORIES:

DINNER

FAT: CARBS: PROTEIN: CALORIES:

SNACKS

FAT: CARBS: PROTEIN: CALORIES:

SLAY the DAY! – MY TOP 6 PRIORITIES

- ○   ○
- ○   ○
- ○   ○

END OF THE DAY TOTAL OVERVIEW

FAT	CARBS	PROTEIN	KCAL

I MAKE PROGRESS EVERY Day

SLEEP TRACKER:

DATE _____

RISE: _____   BEDTIME: _____   SLEEP (HRS): _____

MY NOTES FOR THE DAY

_____
_____
_____

FASTING TIMES & DURATION

EXERCISE / WORKOUT ROUTINE

SLAY the DAY! – MY TOP 6 PRIORITIES

- ○ _____   ○ _____
- ○ _____   ○ _____
- ○ _____   ○ _____

IN A STATE OF KETOSIS?

YES   NO   UNSURE

WATER INTAKE TRACKER

DAILY ENERGY LEVEL

F*CKING GREAT   OKAY   SH*TTY

BREAKFAST

FAT: CARBS: PROTEIN: CALORIES:

LUNCH

FAT: CARBS: PROTEIN: CALORIES:

DINNER

FAT: CARBS: PROTEIN: CALORIES:

SNACKS

FAT: CARBS: PROTEIN: CALORIES:

END OF THE DAY TOTAL OVERVIEW

FAT	CARBS	PROTEIN	KCAL

MEAL **Planner**

WEEK OF

GROCERY LIST

- [ ]
- [ ]
- [ ]
- [ ]
- [ ]
- [ ]
- [ ]
- [ ]
- [ ]
- [ ]
- [ ]
- [ ]
- [ ]
- [ ]
- [ ]
- [ ]
- [ ]

MON

TUES

WED

THUR

FRI

SAT

SUN

Low Carb Shopping List

FRESH PRODUCE

MEAT AND SEAFOOD

DAIRY PRODUCTS

PANTRY ITEMS

FROZEN / OTHER

I MAKE PROGRESS EVERY Day

SLEEP TRACKER:

DATE _____

☼ RISE: _____

🌙 zᶻᶻ BEDTIME: _____

💭zᶻᶻ SLEEP (HRS): _____

MY NOTES FOR THE DAY

_____

_____

_____

FASTING TIMES & DURATION

EXERCISE / WORKOUT ROUTINE

SLAY the DAY! – MY TOP 6 PRIORITIES

IN A STATE OF KETOSIS?

YES   NO   UNSURE

WATER INTAKE TRACKER

💧 💧 💧 💧 💧 💧 💧 💧

DAILY ENERGY LEVEL		
F*CKING GREAT	OKAY	SH*TTY

BREAKFAST

FAT: CARBS: PROTEIN: CALORIES:

LUNCH

FAT: CARBS: PROTEIN: CALORIES:

DINNER

FAT: CARBS: PROTEIN: CALORIES:

SNACKS

FAT: CARBS: PROTEIN: CALORIES:

END OF THE DAY TOTAL OVERVIEW

FAT	CARBS	PROTEIN	KCAL

I MAKE PROGRESS EVERY Day

SLEEP TRACKER:

DATE _____

☀ RISE: _____   🌙 BEDTIME: _____   💤 SLEEP (HRS): _____

MY NOTES FOR THE DAY

_____

_____

_____

FASTING TIMES & DURATION

EXERCISE / WORKOUT ROUTINE

SLAY the DAY! – MY TOP 6 PRIORITIES

- ⚬ _____   ⚬ _____
- ⚬ _____   ⚬ _____
- ⚬ _____   ⚬ _____

IN A STATE OF KETOSIS?

YES   NO   UNSURE

WATER INTAKE TRACKER

DAILY ENERGY LEVEL

F*CKING GREAT   OKAY   SH*TTY

BREAKFAST

FAT: CARBS: PROTEIN: CALORIES:

LUNCH

FAT: CARBS: PROTEIN: CALORIES:

DINNER

FAT: CARBS: PROTEIN: CALORIES:

SNACKS

FAT: CARBS: PROTEIN: CALORIES:

END OF THE DAY TOTAL OVERVIEW

FAT	CARBS	PROTEIN	KCAL

I MAKE PROGRESS EVERY **Day**

SLEEP TRACKER:

DATE _____

☼ | RISE: | 🌙 | BEDTIME: | 💤 | SLEEP (HRS): |

MY NOTES FOR THE DAY

_____

_____

_____

FASTING TIMES & DURATION

EXERCISE / WORKOUT ROUTINE

SLAY the DAY! – MY TOP 6 PRIORITIES

○ _____   ○ _____
○ _____   ○ _____
○ _____   ○ _____

IN A STATE OF KETOSIS?

YES   NO   UNSURE

WATER INTAKE TRACKER

💧 💧 💧 💧 💧 💧 💧 💧

DAILY ENERGY LEVEL
F*CKING GREAT   OKAY   SH*TTY

BREAKFAST

FAT: CARBS: PROTEIN: CALORIES:

LUNCH

FAT: CARBS: PROTEIN: CALORIES:

DINNER

FAT: CARBS: PROTEIN: CALORIES:

SNACKS

FAT: CARBS: PROTEIN: CALORIES:

END OF THE DAY TOTAL OVERVIEW

FAT   CARBS   PROTEIN   KCAL

_____   _____   _____   _____

I MAKE PROGRESS EVERY **Day**

SLEEP TRACKER:

DATE _____

RISE: _____   BEDTIME: _____   SLEEP (HRS): _____

MY NOTES FOR THE DAY	IN A STATE OF KETOSIS?

_____

_____

_____

YES   NO   UNSURE

WATER INTAKE TRACKER

FASTING TIMES & DURATION

DAILY ENERGY LEVEL

F*CKING GREAT	OKAY	SH*TTY

BREAKFAST

FAT: CARBS: PROTEIN: CALORIES:

LUNCH

FAT: CARBS: PROTEIN: CALORIES:

EXERCISE / WORKOUT ROUTINE

DINNER

FAT: CARBS: PROTEIN: CALORIES:

SNACKS

FAT: CARBS: PROTEIN: CALORIES:

SLAY the DAY! – MY TOP 6 PRIORITIES

END OF THE DAY TOTAL OVERVIEW

FAT	CARBS	PROTEIN	KCAL

I MAKE PROGRESS EVERY Day

SLEEP TRACKER:

DATE _____

RISE: _____   BEDTIME: _____   SLEEP (HRS): _____

MY NOTES FOR THE DAY

_____
_____
_____

FASTING TIMES & DURATION

EXERCISE / WORKOUT ROUTINE

SLAY the DAY! – MY TOP 6 PRIORITIES

- ○ _____   ○ _____
- ○ _____   ○ _____
- ○ _____   ○ _____

IN A STATE OF KETOSIS?

YES   NO   UNSURE

WATER INTAKE TRACKER

DAILY ENERGY LEVEL

F*CKING GREAT   OKAY   SH*TTY

BREAKFAST

FAT: CARBS: PROTEIN: CALORIES:

LUNCH

FAT: CARBS: PROTEIN: CALORIES:

DINNER

FAT: CARBS: PROTEIN: CALORIES:

SNACKS

FAT: CARBS: PROTEIN: CALORIES:

END OF THE DAY TOTAL OVERVIEW

FAT	CARBS	PROTEIN	KCAL

I MAKE PROGRESS EVERY Day

SLEEP TRACKER:

DATE _____

RISE: _____   BEDTIME: _____   SLEEP (HRS): _____

MY NOTES FOR THE DAY

_____

_____

_____

IN A STATE OF KETOSIS?

YES   NO   UNSURE

WATER INTAKE TRACKER

FASTING TIMES & DURATION

DAILY ENERGY LEVEL

F*CKING GREAT   OKAY   SH*TTY

BREAKFAST

FAT: CARBS: PROTEIN: CALORIES:

LUNCH

FAT: CARBS: PROTEIN: CALORIES:

EXERCISE / WORKOUT ROUTINE

DINNER

FAT: CARBS: PROTEIN: CALORIES:

SNACKS

FAT: CARBS: PROTEIN: CALORIES:

SLAY the DAY! – MY TOP 6 PRIORITIES

END OF THE DAY TOTAL OVERVIEW

FAT   CARBS   PROTEIN   KCAL

I MAKE PROGRESS EVERY **Day**

SLEEP TRACKER:

DATE _____

☼ RISE: _____   🌙 z z z BEDTIME: _____   💤 z z z SLEEP (HRS): _____

MY NOTES FOR THE DAY

_____
_____
_____

FASTING TIMES & DURATION

EXERCISE / WORKOUT ROUTINE

SLAY the DAY! – MY TOP 6 PRIORITIES

- ○ _____   ○ _____
- ○ _____   ○ _____
- ○ _____   ○ _____

IN A STATE OF KETOSIS?

YES   NO   UNSURE

WATER INTAKE TRACKER

DAILY ENERGY LEVEL

F*CKING GREAT	OKAY	SH*TTY

BREAKFAST

FAT: CARBS: PROTEIN: CALORIES:

LUNCH

FAT: CARBS: PROTEIN: CALORIES:

DINNER

FAT: CARBS: PROTEIN: CALORIES:

SNACKS

FAT: CARBS: PROTEIN: CALORIES:

END OF THE DAY TOTAL OVERVIEW

FAT	CARBS	PROTEIN	KCAL

MEAL **Planner**

GROCERY LIST

- [ ]
- [ ]
- [ ]
- [ ]
- [ ]
- [ ]
- [ ]
- [ ]
- [ ]
- [ ]
- [ ]
- [ ]
- [ ]
- [ ]
- [ ]
- [ ]
- [ ]
- [ ]
- [ ]

MON

TUES

WED

THUR

FRI

SAT

SUN

Low Carb Shopping List

FRESH PRODUCE

MEAT AND SEAFOOD

DAIRY PRODUCTS

PANTRY ITEMS

FROZEN / OTHER

I MAKE PROGRESS EVERY **Day**

SLEEP TRACKER:

DATE _____

RISE: _____   BEDTIME: _____   SLEEP (HRS): _____

MY NOTES FOR THE DAY

_____

_____

_____

FASTING TIMES & DURATION

EXERCISE / WORKOUT ROUTINE

SLAY the DAY! – MY TOP 6 PRIORITIES

- ○ _____   ○ _____
- ○ _____   ○ _____
- ○ _____   ○ _____

IN A STATE OF KETOSIS?

YES   NO   UNSURE

WATER INTAKE TRACKER

DAILY ENERGY LEVEL

F*CKING GREAT	OKAY	SH*TTY

BREAKFAST

FAT: CARBS: PROTEIN: CALORIES:

LUNCH

FAT: CARBS: PROTEIN: CALORIES:

DINNER

FAT: CARBS: PROTEIN: CALORIES:

SNACKS

FAT: CARBS: PROTEIN: CALORIES:

END OF THE DAY TOTAL OVERVIEW

FAT	CARBS	PROTEIN	KCAL

I MAKE PROGRESS EVERY **Day**

DATE _____

RISE: _____   BEDTIME: _____   SLEEP (HRS): _____

MY NOTES FOR THE DAY

_____
_____
_____

IN A STATE OF KETOSIS?

YES   NO   UNSURE

WATER INTAKE TRACKER

FASTING TIMES & DURATION

DAILY ENERGY LEVEL

F*CKING GREAT   OKAY   SH*TTY

BREAKFAST

FAT: CARBS: PROTEIN: CALORIES:

LUNCH

FAT: CARBS: PROTEIN: CALORIES:

EXERCISE / WORKOUT ROUTINE

DINNER

FAT: CARBS: PROTEIN: CALORIES:

SNACKS

FAT: CARBS: PROTEIN: CALORIES:

SLAY the DAY! – MY TOP 6 PRIORITIES

END OF THE DAY TOTAL OVERVIEW

FAT	CARBS	PROTEIN	KCAL

I MAKE PROGRESS EVERY **Day**

DATE _____

RISE: _____   BEDTIME: _____   SLEEP (HRS): _____

MY NOTES FOR THE DAY

_____

_____

_____

FASTING TIMES & DURATION

EXERCISE / WORKOUT ROUTINE

SLAY the DAY! – MY TOP 6 PRIORITIES

- ⦿ _____   ⦿ _____
- ⦿ _____   ⦿ _____
- ⦿ _____   ⦿ _____

IN A STATE OF KETOSIS?

YES   NO   UNSURE

WATER INTAKE TRACKER

DAILY ENERGY LEVEL

F*CKING GREAT   OKAY   SH*TTY

BREAKFAST

FAT: CARBS: PROTEIN: CALORIES:

LUNCH

FAT: CARBS: PROTEIN: CALORIES:

DINNER

FAT: CARBS: PROTEIN: CALORIES:

SNACKS

FAT: CARBS: PROTEIN: CALORIES:

END OF THE DAY TOTAL OVERVIEW

FAT	CARBS	PROTEIN	KCAL

I MAKE PROGRESS EVERY **Day**

SLEEP TRACKER:

DATE _____

RISE: _____

BEDTIME: _____

SLEEP (HRS): _____

MY NOTES FOR THE DAY

_____
_____
_____

FASTING TIMES & DURATION

EXERCISE / WORKOUT ROUTINE

SLAY the DAY! – MY TOP 6 PRIORITIES

- ○ _____ ○ _____
- ○ _____ ○ _____
- ○ _____ ○ _____

IN A STATE OF KETOSIS?

YES   NO   UNSURE

WATER INTAKE TRACKER

DAILY ENERGY LEVEL

F*CKING GREAT   OKAY   SH*TTY

BREAKFAST

FAT: CARBS: PROTEIN: CALORIES:

LUNCH

FAT: CARBS: PROTEIN: CALORIES:

DINNER

FAT: CARBS: PROTEIN: CALORIES:

SNACKS

FAT: CARBS: PROTEIN: CALORIES:

END OF THE DAY TOTAL OVERVIEW

FAT	CARBS	PROTEIN	KCAL

I MAKE PROGRESS EVERY **Day**

SLEEP TRACKER:

DATE _____

RISE: _____   BEDTIME: _____   SLEEP (HRS): _____

MY NOTES FOR THE DAY

_____
_____
_____

FASTING TIMES & DURATION

EXERCISE / WORKOUT ROUTINE

SLAY the DAY! – MY TOP 6 PRIORITIES

- ○ _____   ○ _____
- ○ _____   ○ _____
- ○ _____   ○ _____

IN A STATE OF KETOSIS?

YES   NO   UNSURE

WATER INTAKE TRACKER

DAILY ENERGY LEVEL

F*CKING GREAT   OKAY   SH*TTY

BREAKFAST

FAT: CARBS: PROTEIN: CALORIES:

LUNCH

FAT: CARBS: PROTEIN: CALORIES:

DINNER

FAT: CARBS: PROTEIN: CALORIES:

SNACKS

FAT: CARBS: PROTEIN: CALORIES:

END OF THE DAY TOTAL OVERVIEW

FAT   CARBS   PROTEIN   KCAL

I MAKE PROGRESS EVERY Day

SLEEP TRACKER:

DATE _____

RISE: _____   BEDTIME: _____   SLEEP (HRS): _____

MY NOTES FOR THE DAY

_____
_____
_____

FASTING TIMES & DURATION

EXERCISE / WORKOUT ROUTINE

SLAY the DAY! – MY TOP 6 PRIORITIES

-
-
-
-
-
-

IN A STATE OF KETOSIS?

YES   NO   UNSURE

WATER INTAKE TRACKER

DAILY ENERGY LEVEL

F*CKING GREAT   OKAY   SH*TTY

BREAKFAST

FAT: CARBS: PROTEIN: CALORIES:

LUNCH

FAT: CARBS: PROTEIN: CALORIES:

DINNER

FAT: CARBS: PROTEIN: CALORIES:

SNACKS

FAT: CARBS: PROTEIN: CALORIES:

END OF THE DAY TOTAL OVERVIEW

FAT	CARBS	PROTEIN	KCAL

I MAKE PROGRESS EVERY **Day**

SLEEP TRACKER:

DATE _____

☀ RISE: _____   🌙 zᶻᶻ BEDTIME: _____   💭 SLEEP (HRS): _____

MY NOTES FOR THE DAY

_____
_____
_____

FASTING TIMES & DURATION

EXERCISE / WORKOUT ROUTINE

SLAY the DAY! – MY TOP 6 PRIORITIES

- ○ _____   ○ _____
- ○ _____   ○ _____
- ○ _____   ○ _____

IN A STATE OF KETOSIS?

YES   NO   UNSURE

WATER INTAKE TRACKER

💧 💧 💧 💧 💧 💧 💧 💧

DAILY ENERGY LEVEL		
F*CKING GREAT	**OKAY**	**SH*TTY**

BREAKFAST

FAT: CARBS: PROTEIN: CALORIES:

LUNCH

FAT: CARBS: PROTEIN: CALORIES:

DINNER

FAT: CARBS: PROTEIN: CALORIES:

SNACKS

FAT: CARBS: PROTEIN: CALORIES:

END OF THE DAY TOTAL OVERVIEW

FAT	CARBS	PROTEIN	KCAL

MEAL **Planner**

GROCERY LIST

MON

TUES

WED

THUR

FRI

SAT

SUN

Low Carb Shopping List

FRESH PRODUCE

MEAT AND SEAFOOD

DAIRY PRODUCTS

PANTRY ITEMS

FROZEN / OTHER

I MAKE PROGRESS EVERY **Day**

SLEEP TRACKER:

DATE _____

RISE: _____   BEDTIME: _____   SLEEP (HRS): _____

MY NOTES FOR THE DAY

_____
_____
_____

FASTING TIMES & DURATION

EXERCISE / WORKOUT ROUTINE

SLAY the DAY! – MY TOP 6 PRIORITIES

-
-
-

IN A STATE OF KETOSIS?

YES   NO   UNSURE

WATER INTAKE TRACKER

DAILY ENERGY LEVEL

F*CKING GREAT	OKAY	SH*TTY

BREAKFAST

FAT: CARBS: PROTEIN: CALORIES:

LUNCH

FAT: CARBS: PROTEIN: CALORIES:

DINNER

FAT: CARBS: PROTEIN: CALORIES:

SNACKS

FAT: CARBS: PROTEIN: CALORIES:

END OF THE DAY TOTAL OVERVIEW

FAT	CARBS	PROTEIN	KCAL

I MAKE PROGRESS EVERY **Day**

SLEEP TRACKER:

DATE _____

☼ | RISE: |) zzz | BEDTIME: | 💭zzz | SLEEP (HRS): |

MY NOTES FOR THE DAY

_____

_____

_____

FASTING TIMES & DURATION

EXERCISE / WORKOUT ROUTINE

SLAY the DAY! – MY TOP 6 PRIORITIES

○ _____ ○ _____

○ _____ ○ _____

○ _____ ○ _____

IN A STATE OF KETOSIS?

YES　　　NO　　　UNSURE

WATER INTAKE TRACKER

💧 💧 💧 💧 💧 💧 💧 💧

DAILY ENERGY LEVEL

F*CKING GREAT　　OKAY　　SH*TTY

BREAKFAST

FAT:　　CARBS:　　PROTEIN:　　CALORIES:

LUNCH

FAT:　　CARBS:　　PROTEIN:　　CALORIES:

DINNER

FAT:　　CARBS:　　PROTEIN:　　CALORIES:

SNACKS

FAT:　　CARBS:　　PROTEIN:　　CALORIES:

END OF THE DAY TOTAL OVERVIEW

FAT　　　CARBS　　　PROTEIN　　　KCAL

I MAKE PROGRESS EVERY **Day**

SLEEP TRACKER:

DATE _____

☀ RISE: _____   🌙 BEDTIME: _____   💤 SLEEP (HRS): _____

MY NOTES FOR THE DAY
_____
_____
_____

FASTING TIMES & DURATION

EXERCISE / WORKOUT ROUTINE

SLAY the DAY! – MY TOP 6 PRIORITIES
- ○
- ○
- ○
- ○
- ○
- ○

IN A STATE OF KETOSIS?

YES   NO   UNSURE

WATER INTAKE TRACKER

💧 💧 💧 💧 💧 💧 💧 💧

DAILY ENERGY LEVEL

F*CKING GREAT   OKAY   SH*TTY

BREAKFAST

FAT: CARBS: PROTEIN: CALORIES:

LUNCH

FAT: CARBS: PROTEIN: CALORIES:

DINNER

FAT: CARBS: PROTEIN: CALORIES:

SNACKS

FAT: CARBS: PROTEIN: CALORIES:

END OF THE DAY TOTAL OVERVIEW

FAT	CARBS	PROTEIN	KCAL

I MAKE PROGRESS EVERY Day

SLEEP TRACKER:

DATE _____

RISE: _____   BEDTIME: _____   SLEEP (HRS): _____

MY NOTES FOR THE DAY

_____
_____
_____

IN A STATE OF KETOSIS?

YES   NO   UNSURE

WATER INTAKE TRACKER

FASTING TIMES & DURATION

DAILY ENERGY LEVEL
F*CKING GREAT   **OKAY**   **SH*TTY**

BREAKFAST

FAT: CARBS: PROTEIN: CALORIES:

EXERCISE / WORKOUT ROUTINE

LUNCH

FAT: CARBS: PROTEIN: CALORIES:

DINNER

FAT: CARBS: PROTEIN: CALORIES:

SNACKS

FAT: CARBS: PROTEIN: CALORIES:

SLAY the DAY! – MY TOP 6 PRIORITIES

END OF THE DAY TOTAL OVERVIEW

FAT   CARBS   PROTEIN   KCAL

I MAKE PROGRESS EVERY **Day**

SLEEP TRACKER:

DATE _____

RISE: _____   BEDTIME: _____   SLEEP (HRS): _____

MY NOTES FOR THE DAY

_____
_____
_____

FASTING TIMES & DURATION

EXERCISE / WORKOUT ROUTINE

SLAY the DAY! – MY TOP 6 PRIORITIES

IN A STATE OF KETOSIS?

YES   NO   UNSURE

WATER INTAKE TRACKER

DAILY ENERGY LEVEL

F*CKING GREAT   OKAY   SH*TTY

BREAKFAST

FAT: CARBS: PROTEIN: CALORIES:

LUNCH

FAT: CARBS: PROTEIN: CALORIES:

DINNER

FAT: CARBS: PROTEIN: CALORIES:

SNACKS

FAT: CARBS: PROTEIN: CALORIES:

END OF THE DAY TOTAL OVERVIEW

FAT   CARBS   PROTEIN   KCAL

I MAKE PROGRESS EVERY Day

SLEEP TRACKER:

DATE _____

RISE: _____ BEDTIME: _____ SLEEP (HRS): _____

MY NOTES FOR THE DAY

_____

_____

_____

FASTING TIMES & DURATION

EXERCISE / WORKOUT ROUTINE

SLAY the DAY! – MY TOP 6 PRIORITIES

○ _____ ○ _____

○ _____ ○ _____

○ _____ ○ _____

IN A STATE OF KETOSIS?

YES   NO   UNSURE

WATER INTAKE TRACKER

DAILY ENERGY LEVEL

F*CKING GREAT   OKAY   SH*TTY

BREAKFAST

FAT: CARBS: PROTEIN: CALORIES:

LUNCH

FAT: CARBS: PROTEIN: CALORIES:

DINNER

FAT: CARBS: PROTEIN: CALORIES:

SNACKS

FAT: CARBS: PROTEIN: CALORIES:

END OF THE DAY TOTAL OVERVIEW

FAT	CARBS	PROTEIN	KCAL

I MAKE PROGRESS EVERY **Day**

SLEEP TRACKER:

DATE _____

RISE: _____

BEDTIME: _____

SLEEP (HRS): _____

MY NOTES FOR THE DAY

_____

_____

_____

FASTING TIMES & DURATION

EXERCISE / WORKOUT ROUTINE

SLAY the DAY! – MY TOP 6 PRIORITIES

-
-
-
-
-
-

IN A STATE OF KETOSIS?

YES   NO   UNSURE

WATER INTAKE TRACKER

DAILY ENERGY LEVEL

F*CKING GREAT	OKAY	SH*TTY

BREAKFAST

FAT: CARBS: PROTEIN: CALORIES:

LUNCH

FAT: CARBS: PROTEIN: CALORIES:

DINNER

FAT: CARBS: PROTEIN: CALORIES:

SNACKS

FAT: CARBS: PROTEIN: CALORIES:

END OF THE DAY TOTAL OVERVIEW

FAT	CARBS	PROTEIN	KCAL

MEAL Planner

WEEK OF

GROCERY LIST

- ☐
- ☐
- ☐
- ☐
- ☐
- ☐
- ☐
- ☐
- ☐
- ☐
- ☐
- ☐
- ☐
- ☐
- ☐
- ☐
- ☐
- ☐

MON

TUES

WED

THUR

FRI

SAT

SUN

Low Carb Shopping List

FRESH PRODUCE

MEAT AND SEAFOOD

DAIRY PRODUCTS

PANTRY ITEMS

FROZEN / OTHER

I MAKE PROGRESS EVERY Day

SLEEP TRACKER:

DATE _____

RISE: _____

BEDTIME: _____

SLEEP (HRS): _____

MY NOTES FOR THE DAY

_____
_____
_____

FASTING TIMES & DURATION

EXERCISE / WORKOUT ROUTINE

SLAY the DAY! – MY TOP 6 PRIORITIES

- _____   - _____
- _____   - _____
- _____   - _____

IN A STATE OF KETOSIS?

YES   NO   UNSURE

WATER INTAKE TRACKER

DAILY ENERGY LEVEL

F*CKING GREAT   OKAY   SH*TTY

BREAKFAST

FAT: CARBS: PROTEIN: CALORIES:

LUNCH

FAT: CARBS: PROTEIN: CALORIES:

DINNER

FAT: CARBS: PROTEIN: CALORIES:

SNACKS

FAT: CARBS: PROTEIN: CALORIES:

END OF THE DAY TOTAL OVERVIEW

FAT	CARBS	PROTEIN	KCAL

I MAKE PROGRESS EVERY **Day**

SLEEP TRACKER:

| RISE: | BEDTIME: | SLEEP (HRS): |

MY NOTES FOR THE DAY

_____

_____

_____

FASTING TIMES & DURATION

EXERCISE / WORKOUT ROUTINE

SLAY the DAY! – MY TOP 6 PRIORITIES

IN A STATE OF KETOSIS?

YES   NO   UNSURE

WATER INTAKE TRACKER

DAILY ENERGY LEVEL

F*CKING GREAT   OKAY   SH*TTY

BREAKFAST

| FAT: | CARBS: | PROTEIN: | CALORIES: |

LUNCH

| FAT: | CARBS: | PROTEIN: | CALORIES: |

DINNER

| FAT: | CARBS: | PROTEIN: | CALORIES: |

SNACKS

| FAT: | CARBS: | PROTEIN: | CALORIES: |

END OF THE DAY TOTAL OVERVIEW

FAT	CARBS	PROTEIN	KCAL

I MAKE PROGRESS EVERY **Day**

SLEEP TRACKER:

DATE _____

☀ RISE: _____   🌙 zᶻᶻ BEDTIME: _____   💭 zᶻz SLEEP (HRS): _____

MY NOTES FOR THE DAY

_____
_____
_____

FASTING TIMES & DURATION

EXERCISE / WORKOUT ROUTINE

SLAY the DAY! – MY TOP 6 PRIORITIES

○ _____   ○ _____
○ _____   ○ _____
○ _____   ○ _____

IN A STATE OF KETOSIS?

YES   NO   UNSURE

WATER INTAKE TRACKER

💧 💧 💧 💧 💧 💧 💧 💧

DAILY ENERGY LEVEL		
F*CKING GREAT	OKAY	SH*TTY

BREAKFAST

FAT: CARBS: PROTEIN: CALORIES:

LUNCH

FAT: CARBS: PROTEIN: CALORIES:

DINNER

FAT: CARBS: PROTEIN: CALORIES:

SNACKS

FAT: CARBS: PROTEIN: CALORIES:

END OF THE DAY TOTAL OVERVIEW

FAT	CARBS	PROTEIN	KCAL

I MAKE PROGRESS EVERY Day

DATE _____

RISE: _____

BEDTIME: _____

SLEEP (HRS): _____

MY NOTES FOR THE DAY

_____
_____
_____

FASTING TIMES & DURATION

EXERCISE / WORKOUT ROUTINE

SLAY the DAY! – MY TOP 6 PRIORITIES

- _____
- _____
- _____

IN A STATE OF KETOSIS?

YES   NO   UNSURE

WATER INTAKE TRACKER

DAILY ENERGY LEVEL

F*CKING GREAT   OKAY   SH*TTY

BREAKFAST

FAT: CARBS: PROTEIN: CALORIES:

LUNCH

FAT: CARBS: PROTEIN: CALORIES:

DINNER

FAT: CARBS: PROTEIN: CALORIES:

SNACKS

FAT: CARBS: PROTEIN: CALORIES:

END OF THE DAY TOTAL OVERVIEW

FAT	CARBS	PROTEIN	KCAL

WEIGHT LOSS **Tracker**

WEEKLY WEIGHT LOSS TRACKER – Let's Get This SH*T Done!

MONTHLY GOAL

DATE:					
BUST					
WAIST					
HIPS					
BICEP					
THIGH					
CALF					
WEIGHT					
TOTAL WEIGHT LOSS >>					

INTERMITTENT Fasting Log

	START TIME	END TIME	TOTAL FAST HRS
M	:	:	:
T	:	:	:
W	:	:	:
T	:	:	:
F	:	:	:
S	:	:	:
S	:	:	:

WEEK OF:

	START TIME	END TIME	TOTAL FAST HRS
M	:	:	:
T	:	:	:
W	:	:	:
T	:	:	:
F	:	:	:
S	:	:	:
S	:	:	:

WEEK OF:

	START TIME	END TIME	TOTAL FAST HRS
M	:	:	:
T	:	:	:
W	:	:	:
T	:	:	:
F	:	:	:
S	:	:	:
S	:	:	:

WEEK OF:

	START TIME	END TIME	TOTAL FAST HRS
M	:	:	:
T	:	:	:
W	:	:	:
T	:	:	:
F	:	:	:
S	:	:	:
S	:	:	:

WEEK OF:

	START TIME	END TIME	TOTAL FAST HRS
M	:	:	:
T	:	:	:
W	:	:	:
T	:	:	:
F	:	:	:
S	:	:	:
S	:	:	:

NOTES & REFLECTIONS

MILESTONES & ACCOMPLISHMENTS

GOALS &
Accomplishments

MONTH | JAN FEB MAR APR MAY JUN JUL AUG SEP OCT NOV DEC

THIS MONTH'S F*CKING GOALS

MY F*CKING ACTION PLAN

M T W T F S S

☐☐☐☐☐☐☐
☐☐☐☐☐☐☐
☐☐☐☐☐☐☐
☐☐☐☐☐☐☐
☐☐☐☐☐☐☐

NOTES:

WEEKLY GOALS

THOUGHTS

MEAL IDEAS:	BREAKFAST	LUNCH	DINNER	SNACKS
M				
T				
W				
T				
F				
S				
S				

I MAKE PROGRESS EVERY Day

SLEEP TRACKER:

DATE _____

RISE: _____   BEDTIME: _____   SLEEP (HRS): _____

MY NOTES FOR THE DAY

_____
_____
_____
_____

FASTING TIMES & DURATION

EXERCISE / WORKOUT ROUTINE

SLAY the DAY! – MY TOP 6 PRIORITIES

- ○
- ○
- ○

- ○
- ○
- ○

IN A STATE OF KETOSIS?

YES   NO   UNSURE

WATER INTAKE TRACKER

DAILY ENERGY LEVEL

F*CKING GREAT	OKAY	SH*TTY

BREAKFAST

FAT: CARBS: PROTEIN: CALORIES:

LUNCH

FAT: CARBS: PROTEIN: CALORIES:

DINNER

FAT: CARBS: PROTEIN: CALORIES:

SNACKS

FAT: CARBS: PROTEIN: CALORIES:

END OF THE DAY TOTAL OVERVIEW

FAT	CARBS	PROTEIN	KCAL

I MAKE PROGRESS EVERY **Day**

SLEEP TRACKER:

DATE _____

☀ RISE: _____ 🌙 BEDTIME: _____ 💤 SLEEP (HRS): _____

MY NOTES FOR THE DAY	IN A STATE OF KETOSIS?

_____

_____

_____

YES   NO   UNSURE

WATER INTAKE TRACKER

💧 💧 💧 💧 💧 💧 💧 💧

FASTING TIMES & DURATION

DAILY ENERGY LEVEL

F*CKING GREAT   OKAY   SH*TTY

BREAKFAST

FAT: CARBS: PROTEIN: CALORIES:

EXERCISE / WORKOUT ROUTINE

LUNCH

FAT: CARBS: PROTEIN: CALORIES:

DINNER

FAT: CARBS: PROTEIN: CALORIES:

SNACKS

FAT: CARBS: PROTEIN: CALORIES:

SLAY the DAY! – MY TOP 6 PRIORITIES

- ⊙ _____ ⊙ _____
- ⊙ _____ ⊙ _____
- ⊙ _____ ⊙ _____

END OF THE DAY TOTAL OVERVIEW

FAT   CARBS   PROTEIN   KCAL

I MAKE PROGRESS EVERY **Day**

SLEEP TRACKER:

DATE _____

RISE: _____   BEDTIME: _____   SLEEP (HRS): _____

MY NOTES FOR THE DAY

_____

_____

_____

FASTING TIMES & DURATION

EXERCISE / WORKOUT ROUTINE

SLAY the DAY! – MY TOP 6 PRIORITIES

IN A STATE OF KETOSIS?

YES   NO   UNSURE

WATER INTAKE TRACKER

DAILY ENERGY LEVEL

F*CKING GREAT	OKAY	SH*TTY

BREAKFAST

FAT: CARBS: PROTEIN: CALORIES:

LUNCH

FAT: CARBS: PROTEIN: CALORIES:

DINNER

FAT: CARBS: PROTEIN: CALORIES:

SNACKS

FAT: CARBS: PROTEIN: CALORIES:

END OF THE DAY TOTAL OVERVIEW

FAT	CARBS	PROTEIN	KCAL

MEAL **Planner**

WEEK OF

GROCERY LIST

MON

TUES

WED

THUR

FRI

SAT

SUN

Low Carb Shopping List

FRESH PRODUCE

MEAT AND SEAFOOD

DAIRY PRODUCTS

PANTRY ITEMS

FROZEN / OTHER

I MAKE PROGRESS EVERY **Day**

SLEEP TRACKER:

DATE _____

☀ | RISE: _____ | 🌙 zᶻᶻ | BEDTIME: _____ | 💭zᶻᶻ | SLEEP (HRS): _____

| MY NOTES FOR THE DAY | IN A STATE OF KETOSIS? |

_____

_____

_____

YES   NO   UNSURE

WATER INTAKE TRACKER

💧 💧 💧 💧 💧 💧 💧 💧

FASTING TIMES & DURATION

DAILY ENERGY LEVEL

F*CKING GREAT   OKAY   SH*TTY

BREAKFAST

FAT: CARBS: PROTEIN: CALORIES:

EXERCISE / WORKOUT ROUTINE

LUNCH

FAT: CARBS: PROTEIN: CALORIES:

DINNER

FAT: CARBS: PROTEIN: CALORIES:

SNACKS

FAT: CARBS: PROTEIN: CALORIES:

SLAY the DAY! – MY TOP 6 PRIORITIES

END OF THE DAY TOTAL OVERVIEW

FAT   CARBS   PROTEIN   KCAL

I MAKE PROGRESS EVERY **Day**

SLEEP TRACKER:

DATE _____

☼- RISE: _____ 🌙 zᶻᶻ BEDTIME: _____ 💭 zᶻᶻ SLEEP (HRS): _____

MY NOTES FOR THE DAY

_____
_____
_____
_____

FASTING TIMES & DURATION

EXERCISE / WORKOUT ROUTINE

SLAY the DAY! – MY TOP 6 PRIORITIES

- ⦾ _____   ⦾ _____
- ⦾ _____   ⦾ _____
- ⦾ _____   ⦾ _____

IN A STATE OF KETOSIS?

YES   NO   UNSURE

WATER INTAKE TRACKER

💧 💧 💧 💧 💧 💧 💧 💧

DAILY ENERGY LEVEL		
F*CKING GREAT	OKAY	SH*TTY

BREAKFAST

FAT: CARBS: PROTEIN: CALORIES:

LUNCH

FAT: CARBS: PROTEIN: CALORIES:

DINNER

FAT: CARBS: PROTEIN: CALORIES:

SNACKS

FAT: CARBS: PROTEIN: CALORIES:

END OF THE DAY TOTAL OVERVIEW

FAT	CARBS	PROTEIN	KCAL

I MAKE PROGRESS EVERY **Day**

SLEEP TRACKER:

DATE _____

RISE: _____   BEDTIME: _____   SLEEP (HRS): _____

MY NOTES FOR THE DAY	IN A STATE OF KETOSIS?

_____

_____

_____

YES   NO   UNSURE

WATER INTAKE TRACKER

FASTING TIMES & DURATION

DAILY ENERGY LEVEL		
F*CKING GREAT	**OKAY**	**SH*TTY**

BREAKFAST

FAT: CARBS: PROTEIN: CALORIES:

EXERCISE / WORKOUT ROUTINE

LUNCH

FAT: CARBS: PROTEIN: CALORIES:

DINNER

FAT: CARBS: PROTEIN: CALORIES:

SNACKS

FAT: CARBS: PROTEIN: CALORIES:

SLAY the DAY! – MY TOP 6 PRIORITIES

END OF THE DAY TOTAL OVERVIEW			
FAT	CARBS	PROTEIN	KCAL

I MAKE PROGRESS EVERY **Day**

SLEEP TRACKER:

DATE _____

RISE: _____   BEDTIME: _____   SLEEP (HRS): _____

MY NOTES FOR THE DAY

_____

_____

_____

FASTING TIMES & DURATION

EXERCISE / WORKOUT ROUTINE

SLAY the DAY! – MY TOP 6 PRIORITIES

- ◦ ◦
- ◦ ◦
- ◦ ◦

IN A STATE OF KETOSIS?

YES   NO   UNSURE

WATER INTAKE TRACKER

DAILY ENERGY LEVEL

F*CKING GREAT	OKAY	SH*TTY

BREAKFAST

FAT: CARBS: PROTEIN: CALORIES:

LUNCH

FAT: CARBS: PROTEIN: CALORIES:

DINNER

FAT: CARBS: PROTEIN: CALORIES:

SNACKS

FAT: CARBS: PROTEIN: CALORIES:

END OF THE DAY TOTAL OVERVIEW

FAT	CARBS	PROTEIN	KCAL

I MAKE PROGRESS EVERY **Day**

SLEEP TRACKER:

DATE _____

☀ RISE: [   ]   🌙 BEDTIME: [   ]   💭 SLEEP (HRS): [   ]

MY NOTES FOR THE DAY

_____
_____
_____

FASTING TIMES & DURATION

[   ]

EXERCISE / WORKOUT ROUTINE

[   ]

SLAY the DAY! – MY TOP 6 PRIORITIES

○ _____   ○ _____
○ _____   ○ _____
○ _____   ○ _____

IN A STATE OF KETOSIS?

YES   NO   UNSURE

WATER INTAKE TRACKER

💧 💧 💧 💧 💧 💧 💧

DAILY ENERGY LEVEL		
F*CKING GREAT	OKAY	SH*TTY

BREAKFAST

FAT: CARBS: PROTEIN: CALORIES:

LUNCH

FAT: CARBS: PROTEIN: CALORIES:

DINNER

FAT: CARBS: PROTEIN: CALORIES:

SNACKS

FAT: CARBS: PROTEIN: CALORIES:

END OF THE DAY TOTAL OVERVIEW

FAT	CARBS	PROTEIN	KCAL
[ ]	[ ]	[ ]	[ ]

I MAKE PROGRESS EVERY **Day**

SLEEP TRACKER:

DATE _____

RISE: _____

BEDTIME: _____

SLEEP (HRS): _____

MY NOTES FOR THE DAY

_____
_____
_____

FASTING TIMES & DURATION

EXERCISE / WORKOUT ROUTINE

SLAY the DAY! – MY TOP 6 PRIORITIES

IN A STATE OF KETOSIS?

YES   NO   UNSURE

WATER INTAKE TRACKER

DAILY ENERGY LEVEL		
F*CKING GREAT	OKAY	SH*TTY

BREAKFAST

FAT: CARBS: PROTEIN: CALORIES:

LUNCH

FAT: CARBS: PROTEIN: CALORIES:

DINNER

FAT: CARBS: PROTEIN: CALORIES:

SNACKS

FAT: CARBS: PROTEIN: CALORIES:

END OF THE DAY TOTAL OVERVIEW

FAT	CARBS	PROTEIN	KCAL

I MAKE PROGRESS EVERY **Day**

SLEEP TRACKER:

DATE _____

RISE: _____   BEDTIME: _____   SLEEP (HRS): _____

MY NOTES FOR THE DAY

_____

_____

_____

FASTING TIMES & DURATION

EXERCISE / WORKOUT ROUTINE

SLAY the DAY! – MY TOP 6 PRIORITIES

○ _____   ○ _____
○ _____   ○ _____
○ _____   ○ _____

IN A STATE OF KETOSIS?

YES   NO   UNSURE

WATER INTAKE TRACKER

DAILY ENERGY LEVEL

F*CKING GREAT   OKAY   SH*TTY

BREAKFAST

FAT: CARBS: PROTEIN: CALORIES:

LUNCH

FAT: CARBS: PROTEIN: CALORIES:

DINNER

FAT: CARBS: PROTEIN: CALORIES:

SNACKS

FAT: CARBS: PROTEIN: CALORIES:

END OF THE DAY TOTAL OVERVIEW

FAT	CARBS	PROTEIN	KCAL

MEAL **Planner**

WEEK OF

GROCERY LIST

- [ ]
- [ ]
- [ ]
- [ ]
- [ ]
- [ ]
- [ ]
- [ ]
- [ ]
- [ ]
- [ ]
- [ ]
- [ ]
- [ ]
- [ ]
- [ ]
- [ ]
- [ ]

MON

TUES

WED

THUR

FRI

SAT

SUN

Low Carb Shopping List

FRESH PRODUCE

MEAT AND SEAFOOD

DAIRY PRODUCTS

PANTRY ITEMS

FROZEN / OTHER

I MAKE PROGRESS EVERY **Day**

SLEEP TRACKER:

DATE _____

RISE: _____ BEDTIME: _____ SLEEP (HRS): _____

MY NOTES FOR THE DAY

_____
_____
_____

FASTING TIMES & DURATION

EXERCISE / WORKOUT ROUTINE

SLAY the DAY! – MY TOP 6 PRIORITIES

IN A STATE OF KETOSIS?

YES   NO   UNSURE

WATER INTAKE TRACKER

DAILY ENERGY LEVEL

F*CKING GREAT   OKAY   SH*TTY

BREAKFAST

FAT: CARBS: PROTEIN: CALORIES:

LUNCH

FAT: CARBS: PROTEIN: CALORIES:

DINNER

FAT: CARBS: PROTEIN: CALORIES:

SNACKS

FAT: CARBS: PROTEIN: CALORIES:

END OF THE DAY TOTAL OVERVIEW

FAT   CARBS   PROTEIN   KCAL

I MAKE PROGRESS EVERY **Day**

SLEEP TRACKER:

DATE _____

☀ RISE: [_____]   🌙 BEDTIME: [_____]   💭 SLEEP (HRS): [_____]

MY NOTES FOR THE DAY

_____

_____

_____

FASTING TIMES & DURATION

EXERCISE / WORKOUT ROUTINE

SLAY the DAY! – MY TOP 6 PRIORITIES

⦿ _____   ⦿ _____

⦿ _____   ⦿ _____

⦿ _____   ⦿ _____

IN A STATE OF KETOSIS?

YES   NO   UNSURE

WATER INTAKE TRACKER

💧 💧 💧 💧 💧 💧 💧 💧

DAILY ENERGY LEVEL

F*CKING GREAT   OKAY   SH*TTY

BREAKFAST

FAT: CARBS: PROTEIN: CALORIES:

LUNCH

FAT: CARBS: PROTEIN: CALORIES:

DINNER

FAT: CARBS: PROTEIN: CALORIES:

SNACKS

FAT: CARBS: PROTEIN: CALORIES:

END OF THE DAY TOTAL OVERVIEW

FAT	CARBS	PROTEIN	KCAL
____	____	____	____

I MAKE PROGRESS EVERY Day

SLEEP TRACKER:

DATE _____

RISE: _____

BEDTIME: _____

SLEEP (HRS): _____

MY NOTES FOR THE DAY

_____
_____
_____
_____

FASTING TIMES & DURATION

EXERCISE / WORKOUT ROUTINE

SLAY the DAY! – MY TOP 6 PRIORITIES

- ○ _____ ○ _____
- ○ _____ ○ _____
- ○ _____ ○ _____

IN A STATE OF KETOSIS?

YES   NO   UNSURE

WATER INTAKE TRACKER

DAILY ENERGY LEVEL

F*CKING GREAT   OKAY   SH*TTY

BREAKFAST

FAT: CARBS: PROTEIN: CALORIES:

LUNCH

FAT: CARBS: PROTEIN: CALORIES:

DINNER

FAT: CARBS: PROTEIN: CALORIES:

SNACKS

FAT: CARBS: PROTEIN: CALORIES:

END OF THE DAY TOTAL OVERVIEW

FAT	CARBS	PROTEIN	KCAL

I MAKE PROGRESS EVERY **Day**

SLEEP TRACKER:

DATE _____

RISE: _____   BEDTIME: _____   SLEEP (HRS): _____

MY NOTES FOR THE DAY

_____

_____

_____

FASTING TIMES & DURATION

EXERCISE / WORKOUT ROUTINE

SLAY the DAY! – MY TOP 6 PRIORITIES

- ○ _____   ○ _____
- ○ _____   ○ _____
- ○ _____   ○ _____

IN A STATE OF KETOSIS?

YES   NO   UNSURE

WATER INTAKE TRACKER

DAILY ENERGY LEVEL

F*CKING GREAT   OKAY   SH*TTY

BREAKFAST

FAT: CARBS: PROTEIN: CALORIES:

LUNCH

FAT: CARBS: PROTEIN: CALORIES:

DINNER

FAT: CARBS: PROTEIN: CALORIES:

SNACKS

FAT: CARBS: PROTEIN: CALORIES:

END OF THE DAY TOTAL OVERVIEW

FAT	CARBS	PROTEIN	KCAL

I MAKE PROGRESS EVERY Day

SLEEP TRACKER:

DATE _____

RISE: _____

BEDTIME: _____

SLEEP (HRS): _____

MY NOTES FOR THE DAY

_____

_____

_____

IN A STATE OF KETOSIS?

YES   NO   UNSURE

WATER INTAKE TRACKER

FASTING TIMES & DURATION

DAILY ENERGY LEVEL		
F*CKING GREAT	OKAY	SH*TTY

BREAKFAST

FAT: CARBS: PROTEIN: CALORIES:

EXERCISE / WORKOUT ROUTINE

LUNCH

FAT: CARBS: PROTEIN: CALORIES:

DINNER

FAT: CARBS: PROTEIN: CALORIES:

SNACKS

FAT: CARBS: PROTEIN: CALORIES:

SLAY the DAY! – MY TOP 6 PRIORITIES

END OF THE DAY TOTAL OVERVIEW

FAT	CARBS	PROTEIN	KCAL

I MAKE PROGRESS EVERY **Day**

SLEEP TRACKER:

DATE _____

☼ | RISE: | 🌙 | BEDTIME: | 💤 | SLEEP (HRS): |

MY NOTES FOR THE DAY

_____
_____
_____

IN A STATE OF KETOSIS?

YES   NO   UNSURE

WATER INTAKE TRACKER

💧 💧 💧 💧 💧 💧 💧 💧

FASTING TIMES & DURATION

DAILY ENERGY LEVEL

F*CKING GREAT   OKAY   SH*TTY

BREAKFAST

FAT: CARBS: PROTEIN: CALORIES:

EXERCISE / WORKOUT ROUTINE

LUNCH

FAT: CARBS: PROTEIN: CALORIES:

DINNER

FAT: CARBS: PROTEIN: CALORIES:

SNACKS

FAT: CARBS: PROTEIN: CALORIES:

SLAY the DAY! – MY TOP 6 PRIORITIES

○ _____   ○ _____
○ _____   ○ _____
○ _____   ○ _____

END OF THE DAY TOTAL OVERVIEW

FAT   CARBS   PROTEIN   KCAL

I MAKE PROGRESS EVERY Day

SLEEP TRACKER:

DATE _____

☼ RISE: _____

🌙 z,z,z BEDTIME: _____

💭zzz SLEEP (HRS): _____

MY NOTES FOR THE DAY

_____

_____

_____

FASTING TIMES & DURATION

EXERCISE / WORKOUT ROUTINE

SLAY the DAY! – MY TOP 6 PRIORITIES

○ _____   ○ _____
○ _____   ○ _____
○ _____   ○ _____

IN A STATE OF KETOSIS?

YES   NO   UNSURE

WATER INTAKE TRACKER

💧 💧 💧 💧 💧 💧 💧 💧

DAILY ENERGY LEVEL

F*CKING GREAT   OKAY   SH*TTY

BREAKFAST

FAT: CARBS: PROTEIN: CALORIES:

LUNCH

FAT: CARBS: PROTEIN: CALORIES:

DINNER

FAT: CARBS: PROTEIN: CALORIES:

SNACKS

FAT: CARBS: PROTEIN: CALORIES:

END OF THE DAY TOTAL OVERVIEW

FAT   CARBS   PROTEIN   KCAL

MEAL Planner

WEEK OF

GROCERY LIST

MON

TUES

WED

THUR

FRI

SAT

SUN

Low Carb Shopping List

FRESH PRODUCE

MEAT AND SEAFOOD

DAIRY PRODUCTS

PANTRY ITEMS

FROZEN / OTHER

I MAKE PROGRESS EVERY **Day**

SLEEP TRACKER:

DATE _____

RISE: _____   BEDTIME: _____   SLEEP (HRS): _____

MY NOTES FOR THE DAY

_____

_____

_____

IN A STATE OF KETOSIS?

YES   NO   UNSURE

WATER INTAKE TRACKER

FASTING TIMES & DURATION

DAILY ENERGY LEVEL

F*CKING GREAT   OKAY   SH*TTY

BREAKFAST

FAT: CARBS: PROTEIN: CALORIES:

EXERCISE / WORKOUT ROUTINE

LUNCH

FAT: CARBS: PROTEIN: CALORIES:

DINNER

FAT: CARBS: PROTEIN: CALORIES:

SNACKS

FAT: CARBS: PROTEIN: CALORIES:

SLAY the DAY! – MY TOP 6 PRIORITIES

END OF THE DAY TOTAL OVERVIEW

FAT   CARBS   PROTEIN   KCAL

I MAKE PROGRESS EVERY **Day**

SLEEP TRACKER:

DATE _____

RISE: _____

BEDTIME: _____

SLEEP (HRS): _____

MY NOTES FOR THE DAY

_____
_____
_____

FASTING TIMES & DURATION

EXERCISE / WORKOUT ROUTINE

IN A STATE OF KETOSIS?

YES   NO   UNSURE

WATER INTAKE TRACKER

DAILY ENERGY LEVEL

F*CKING GREAT   OKAY   SH*TTY

BREAKFAST

FAT: CARBS: PROTEIN: CALORIES:

LUNCH

FAT: CARBS: PROTEIN: CALORIES:

DINNER

FAT: CARBS: PROTEIN: CALORIES:

SNACKS

FAT: CARBS: PROTEIN: CALORIES:

SLAY the DAY! – MY TOP 6 PRIORITIES

END OF THE DAY TOTAL OVERVIEW

FAT   CARBS   PROTEIN   KCAL

I MAKE PROGRESS EVERY **Day**

SLEEP TRACKER:

DATE _____

RISE: _____   BEDTIME: _____   SLEEP (HRS): _____

MY NOTES FOR THE DAY

_____
_____
_____

FASTING TIMES & DURATION

EXERCISE / WORKOUT ROUTINE

SLAY the DAY! – MY TOP 6 PRIORITIES

- _____   _____
- _____   _____
- _____   _____

IN A STATE OF KETOSIS?

YES   NO   UNSURE

WATER INTAKE TRACKER

DAILY ENERGY LEVEL

F*CKING GREAT   OKAY   SH*TTY

BREAKFAST

FAT: CARBS: PROTEIN: CALORIES:

LUNCH

FAT: CARBS: PROTEIN: CALORIES:

DINNER

FAT: CARBS: PROTEIN: CALORIES:

SNACKS

FAT: CARBS: PROTEIN: CALORIES:

END OF THE DAY TOTAL OVERVIEW

FAT   CARBS   PROTEIN   KCAL

I MAKE PROGRESS EVERY **Day**

DATE _____

RISE: _____

BEDTIME: _____

SLEEP (HRS): _____

MY NOTES FOR THE DAY

_____
_____
_____

IN A STATE OF KETOSIS?

YES   NO   UNSURE

WATER INTAKE TRACKER

FASTING TIMES & DURATION

DAILY ENERGY LEVEL

F*CKING GREAT	OKAY	SH*TTY

BREAKFAST

FAT: CARBS: PROTEIN: CALORIES:

LUNCH

FAT: CARBS: PROTEIN: CALORIES:

EXERCISE / WORKOUT ROUTINE

DINNER

FAT: CARBS: PROTEIN: CALORIES:

SNACKS

FAT: CARBS: PROTEIN: CALORIES:

SLAY the DAY! – MY TOP 6 PRIORITIES

END OF THE DAY TOTAL OVERVIEW

FAT	CARBS	PROTEIN	KCAL

I MAKE PROGRESS EVERY Day

SLEEP TRACKER:

DATE _____

RISE: _____

BEDTIME: _____

SLEEP (HRS): _____

MY NOTES FOR THE DAY

_____

_____

_____

IN A STATE OF KETOSIS?

YES   NO   UNSURE

WATER INTAKE TRACKER

FASTING TIMES & DURATION

DAILY ENERGY LEVEL

F*CKING GREAT   OKAY   SH*TTY

BREAKFAST

FAT: CARBS: PROTEIN: CALORIES:

EXERCISE / WORKOUT ROUTINE

LUNCH

FAT: CARBS: PROTEIN: CALORIES:

DINNER

FAT: CARBS: PROTEIN: CALORIES:

SNACKS

FAT: CARBS: PROTEIN: CALORIES:

SLAY the DAY! – MY TOP 6 PRIORITIES

END OF THE DAY TOTAL OVERVIEW

FAT   CARBS   PROTEIN   KCAL

I MAKE PROGRESS EVERY **Day**

SLEEP TRACKER:

DATE _____

☼ RISE: _____

🌙 BEDTIME: _____

💤 SLEEP (HRS): _____

MY NOTES FOR THE DAY

_____
_____
_____

FASTING TIMES & DURATION

EXERCISE / WORKOUT ROUTINE

SLAY the DAY! – MY TOP 6 PRIORITIES

IN A STATE OF KETOSIS?

YES   NO   UNSURE

WATER INTAKE TRACKER

DAILY ENERGY LEVEL

F*CKING GREAT	OKAY	SH*TTY

BREAKFAST

FAT: CARBS: PROTEIN: CALORIES:

LUNCH

FAT: CARBS: PROTEIN: CALORIES:

DINNER

FAT: CARBS: PROTEIN: CALORIES:

SNACKS

FAT: CARBS: PROTEIN: CALORIES:

END OF THE DAY TOTAL OVERVIEW

FAT	CARBS	PROTEIN	KCAL

I MAKE PROGRESS EVERY **Day**

SLEEP TRACKER:

DATE _____

☀ RISE: _____ 🌙 BEDTIME: _____ 💭 SLEEP (HRS): _____

MY NOTES FOR THE DAY
_____
_____
_____

IN A STATE OF KETOSIS?

YES   NO   UNSURE

WATER INTAKE TRACKER

💧 💧 💧 💧 💧 💧 💧 💧

FASTING TIMES & DURATION

DAILY ENERGY LEVEL

F*CKING GREAT   OKAY   SH*TTY

BREAKFAST

FAT: CARBS: PROTEIN: CALORIES:

EXERCISE / WORKOUT ROUTINE

LUNCH

FAT: CARBS: PROTEIN: CALORIES:

DINNER

FAT: CARBS: PROTEIN: CALORIES:

SNACKS

FAT: CARBS: PROTEIN: CALORIES:

SLAY the DAY! – MY TOP 6 PRIORITIES

⦿ _____   ⦿ _____
⦿ _____   ⦿ _____
⦿ _____   ⦿ _____

END OF THE DAY TOTAL OVERVIEW

FAT	CARBS	PROTEIN	KCAL

MEAL **Planner**

GROCERY LIST

☐
☐
☐
☐
☐
☐
☐
☐
☐
☐
☐
☐
☐
☐
☐
☐
☐
☐

MON

TUES

WED

THUR

FRI

SAT

SUN

Low Carb Shopping List

FRESH PRODUCE

MEAT AND SEAFOOD

DAIRY PRODUCTS

PANTRY ITEMS

FROZEN / OTHER

I MAKE PROGRESS EVERY **Day**

DATE _____

RISE: _____

BEDTIME: _____

SLEEP (HRS): _____

MY NOTES FOR THE DAY

_____

_____

_____

FASTING TIMES & DURATION

EXERCISE / WORKOUT ROUTINE

SLAY the DAY! – MY TOP 6 PRIORITIES

IN A STATE OF KETOSIS?

YES   NO   UNSURE

WATER INTAKE TRACKER

DAILY ENERGY LEVEL

F*CKING GREAT   OKAY   SH*TTY

BREAKFAST

FAT: CARBS: PROTEIN: CALORIES:

LUNCH

FAT: CARBS: PROTEIN: CALORIES:

DINNER

FAT: CARBS: PROTEIN: CALORIES:

SNACKS

FAT: CARBS: PROTEIN: CALORIES:

END OF THE DAY TOTAL OVERVIEW

FAT   CARBS   PROTEIN   KCAL

I MAKE PROGRESS EVERY **Day**

SLEEP TRACKER:

DATE _____

-Ö- RISE: _____   🌙 BEDTIME: _____   💤 SLEEP (HRS): _____

MY NOTES FOR THE DAY

_____

_____

_____

FASTING TIMES & DURATION

EXERCISE / WORKOUT ROUTINE

SLAY the DAY! – MY TOP 6 PRIORITIES

○ _____   ○ _____

○ _____   ○ _____

○ _____   ○ _____

IN A STATE OF KETOSIS?

YES   NO   UNSURE

WATER INTAKE TRACKER

💧 💧 💧 💧 💧 💧 💧 💧

DAILY ENERGY LEVEL		
F*CKING GREAT	OKAY	SH*TTY

BREAKFAST

FAT: CARBS: PROTEIN: CALORIES:

LUNCH

FAT: CARBS: PROTEIN: CALORIES:

DINNER

FAT: CARBS: PROTEIN: CALORIES:

SNACKS

FAT: CARBS: PROTEIN: CALORIES:

END OF THE DAY TOTAL OVERVIEW

FAT	CARBS	PROTEIN	KCAL

I MAKE PROGRESS EVERY Day

SLEEP TRACKER:

DATE _____

☀ RISE: _____   🌙 BEDTIME: _____   💤 SLEEP (HRS): _____

MY NOTES FOR THE DAY	IN A STATE OF KETOSIS?

_____

_____

_____

IN A STATE OF KETOSIS?

YES   NO   UNSURE

WATER INTAKE TRACKER

💧 💧 💧 💧 💧 💧 💧 💧

FASTING TIMES & DURATION

DAILY ENERGY LEVEL

F*CKING GREAT   OKAY   SH*TTY

BREAKFAST

FAT: CARBS: PROTEIN: CALORIES:

EXERCISE / WORKOUT ROUTINE

LUNCH

FAT: CARBS: PROTEIN: CALORIES:

DINNER

FAT: CARBS: PROTEIN: CALORIES:

SNACKS

FAT: CARBS: PROTEIN: CALORIES:

SLAY the DAY! – MY TOP 6 PRIORITIES

- ○ _____   ○ _____
- ○ _____   ○ _____
- ○ _____   ○ _____

END OF THE DAY TOTAL OVERVIEW

FAT	CARBS	PROTEIN	KCAL

I MAKE PROGRESS EVERY **Day**

SLEEP TRACKER:

DATE _____

☀ RISE: _____   🌙 zzz BEDTIME: _____   💭zzz SLEEP (HRS): _____

MY NOTES FOR THE DAY

_____

_____

_____

FASTING TIMES & DURATION

EXERCISE / WORKOUT ROUTINE

SLAY the DAY! – MY TOP 6 PRIORITIES

◉ _____   ◉ _____

◉ _____   ◉ _____

◉ _____   ◉ _____

IN A STATE OF KETOSIS?

YES   NO   UNSURE

WATER INTAKE TRACKER

💧 💧 💧 💧 💧 💧 💧 💧

DAILY ENERGY LEVEL		
F*CKING GREAT	OKAY	SH*TTY

BREAKFAST

FAT: CARBS: PROTEIN: CALORIES:

LUNCH

FAT: CARBS: PROTEIN: CALORIES:

DINNER

FAT: CARBS: PROTEIN: CALORIES:

SNACKS

FAT: CARBS: PROTEIN: CALORIES:

END OF THE DAY TOTAL OVERVIEW

FAT	CARBS	PROTEIN	KCAL

I MAKE PROGRESS EVERY Day

SLEEP TRACKER:

DATE _____

☀ RISE: _____

🌙 zzz BEDTIME: _____

💤 SLEEP (HRS): _____

MY NOTES FOR THE DAY

_____

_____

_____

FASTING TIMES & DURATION

EXERCISE / WORKOUT ROUTINE

SLAY the DAY! – MY TOP 6 PRIORITIES

- ○ _____   ○ _____
- ○ _____   ○ _____
- ○ _____   ○ _____

IN A STATE OF KETOSIS?

YES   NO   UNSURE

WATER INTAKE TRACKER

💧 💧 💧 💧 💧 💧 💧 💧

DAILY ENERGY LEVEL

F*CKING GREAT   OKAY   SH*TTY

BREAKFAST

FAT: CARBS: PROTEIN: CALORIES:

LUNCH

FAT: CARBS: PROTEIN: CALORIES:

DINNER

FAT: CARBS: PROTEIN: CALORIES:

SNACKS

FAT: CARBS: PROTEIN: CALORIES:

END OF THE DAY TOTAL OVERVIEW

FAT	CARBS	PROTEIN	KCAL

I MAKE PROGRESS EVERY **Day**

SLEEP TRACKER:

DATE _____

RISE: _____

BEDTIME: _____

SLEEP (HRS): _____

MY NOTES FOR THE DAY	IN A STATE OF KETOSIS?

_____

_____

_____

IN A STATE OF KETOSIS?

YES   NO   UNSURE

WATER INTAKE TRACKER

FASTING TIMES & DURATION

DAILY ENERGY LEVEL

F*CKING GREAT   OKAY   SH*TTY

BREAKFAST

FAT: CARBS: PROTEIN: CALORIES:

EXERCISE / WORKOUT ROUTINE

LUNCH

FAT: CARBS: PROTEIN: CALORIES:

DINNER

FAT: CARBS: PROTEIN: CALORIES:

SNACKS

FAT: CARBS: PROTEIN: CALORIES:

SLAY the DAY! – MY TOP 6 PRIORITIES

END OF THE DAY TOTAL OVERVIEW

FAT   CARBS   PROTEIN   KCAL

I MAKE PROGRESS EVERY Day

SLEEP TRACKER:

DATE _____

RISE: _____

BEDTIME: _____

SLEEP (HRS): _____

MY NOTES FOR THE DAY

_____
_____
_____

FASTING TIMES & DURATION

EXERCISE / WORKOUT ROUTINE

SLAY the DAY! – MY TOP 6 PRIORITIES

- ⦾ _____   ⦾ _____
- ⦾ _____   ⦾ _____
- ⦾ _____   ⦾ _____

IN A STATE OF KETOSIS?

YES   NO   UNSURE

WATER INTAKE TRACKER

DAILY ENERGY LEVEL

F*CKING GREAT   OKAY   SH*TTY

BREAKFAST

FAT: CARBS: PROTEIN: CALORIES:

LUNCH

FAT: CARBS: PROTEIN: CALORIES:

DINNER

FAT: CARBS: PROTEIN: CALORIES:

SNACKS

FAT: CARBS: PROTEIN: CALORIES:

END OF THE DAY TOTAL OVERVIEW

FAT	CARBS	PROTEIN	KCAL

WEIGHT LOSS End Date

What are some of my thoughts about my 90-Day Keto Journey? How the hell did it go?

Will I continue to do Keto? What the hell will I do differently? What kind of sh*t will I do more of?

PERSONAL MILESTONES

WEIGHT LOSS **Results**

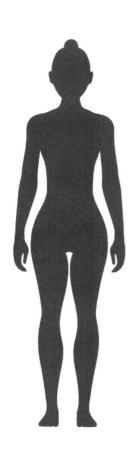

DATE: _____

CHEST	
WAIST	
SHOULDERS	
UPPER ARM	
FOREARM	
CALF	
WEIGHT	
TOTAL WEIGHT LOSS >>	

DAMN GOOD KETO Recipe

RECIPE NAME:

	Keto	Low Carb	Paleo	Vegetarian	Vegan	Dairy Free	Gluten Free
	☐	☐	☐	☐	☐	☐	☐

QTY	INGREDIENTS	RECIPE INSTRUCTIONS

NOTES & RECIPE REVIEW		Serves	
		Prep Time	
		Cook Time	
		Tools	
		Temp	

Total	Carbs	Fat	Protein	Cals

DAMN GOOD KETO **Recipe**

RECIPE NAME:

	Keto	Low Carb	Paleo	Vegetarian	Vegan	Dairy Free	Gluten Free
	☐	☐	☐	☐	☐	☐	☐

QTY	INGREDIENTS

RECIPE INSTRUCTIONS

NOTES & RECIPE REVIEW

Serves	
Prep Time	
Cook Time	
Tools	
Temp	

Total	Carbs	Fat	Protein	Cals

DAMN GOOD KETO **Recipe**

RECIPE NAME:

_____

Keto	Low Carb	Paleo	Vegetarian	Vegan	Dairy Free	Gluten Free
☐	☐	☐	☐	☐	☐	☐

QTY	INGREDIENTS	RECIPE INSTRUCTIONS

NOTES & RECIPE REVIEW		Serves	
		Prep Time	
		Cook Time	
		Tools	
		Temp	

		Carbs	Fat	Protein	Cals
Total					

DAMN GOOD KETO **Recipe**

RECIPE NAME:

	Keto	Low Carb	Paleo	Vegetarian	Vegan	Dairy Free	Gluten Free
	☐	☐	☐	☐	☐	☐	☐

QTY	INGREDIENTS	RECIPE INSTRUCTIONS

NOTES & RECIPE REVIEW

Serves	
Prep Time	
Cook Time	
Tools	
Temp	

Total	Carbs	Fat	Protein	Cals

DAMN GOOD KETO **Recipe**

RECIPE NAME:

_____

Keto	Low Carb	Paleo	Vegetarian	Vegan	Dairy Free	Gluten Free
☐	☐	☐	☐	☐	☐	☐

QTY	INGREDIENTS	RECIPE INSTRUCTIONS

NOTES & RECIPE REVIEW		Serves	
		Prep Time	
		Cook Time	
		Tools	
		Temp	

Total	Carbs	Fat	Protein	Cals

DAMN GOOD KETO **Recipe**

RECIPE NAME:
_____

	Keto	Low Carb	Paleo	Vegetarian	Vegan	Dairy Free	Gluten Free
	☐	☐	☐	☐	☐	☐	☐

QTY	INGREDIENTS	RECIPE INSTRUCTIONS

NOTES & RECIPE REVIEW

Serves	
Prep Time	
Cook Time	
Tools	
Temp	

Total	Carbs	Fat	Protein	Cals

DAMN GOOD KETO Recipe

RECIPE NAME:

_____

Keto	Low Carb	Paleo	Vegetarian	Vegan	Dairy Free	Gluten Free
☐	☐	☐	☐	☐	☐	☐

QTY	INGREDIENTS	RECIPE INSTRUCTIONS

NOTES & RECIPE REVIEW

Serves	
Prep Time	
Cook Time	
Tools	
Temp	

Total	Carbs	Fat	Protein	Cals

DAMN GOOD KETO **Recipe**

RECIPE NAME:

	Keto	Low Carb	Paleo	Vegetarian	Vegan	Dairy Free	Gluten Free
	☐	☐	☐	☐	☐	☐	☐

QTY	INGREDIENTS	RECIPE INSTRUCTIONS

NOTES & RECIPE REVIEW		
	Serves	
	Prep Time	
	Cook Time	
	Tools	
	Temp	

Total	Carbs	Fat	Protein	Cals

DAMN GOOD KETO **Recipe**

RECIPE NAME:

_____

Keto	Low Carb	Paleo	Vegetarian	Vegan	Dairy Free	Gluten Free
☐	☐	☐	☐	☐	☐	☐

QTY	INGREDIENTS	RECIPE INSTRUCTIONS

NOTES & RECIPE REVIEW

Serves	
Prep Time	
Cook Time	
Tools	
Temp	

Total	Carbs	Fat	Protein	Cals

DAMN GOOD KETO **Recipe**

RECIPE NAME:

_____

	Keto	Low Carb	Paleo	Vegetarian	Vegan	Dairy Free	Gluten Free
	☐	☐	☐	☐	☐	☐	☐

QTY	INGREDIENTS	RECIPE INSTRUCTIONS

NOTES & RECIPE REVIEW

Serves	
Prep Time	
Cook Time	
Tools	
Temp	

Total	Carbs	Fat	Protein	Cals

Made in the USA
Monee, IL
10 November 2020

47210912R00085